OWEN HUNTER

Jessner's Lymphocytic Infiltrate

Your Comprehensive Blueprint for Diagnosis and Treatment

First edition

This book was professionally typeset on Reedsy.
Find out more at reedsy.com

Contents

INTRODUCTION

Introduction to Jessner's Lymphocytic Infiltrate

In the vast landscape of dermatological conditions, Jessner's Lymphocytic Infiltrate (JLI) stands as a fascinating yet often misunderstood entity. Named after the German-American dermatologist Max Jessner, who first described it in collaboration with his colleague Norman Kanof in 1953, this condition has intrigued and challenged medical professionals for decades. As we embark on this comprehensive exploration of JLI, we find ourselves at the intersection of dermatology, immunology, and patient care, navigating a condition that exemplifies the complexities of skin disorders and the immune system's role in cutaneous health.

Jessner's Lymphocytic Infiltrate, also known as Jessner's lymphocytic infiltration of the skin or Jessner-Kanof syndrome, is characterized by the appearance of erythematous papules or plaques, typically on the face, neck, and upper back. These lesions, while benign, can be persistent and psychologically distressing for those affected. The hallmark of JLI is a dense infiltrate of lymphocytes in the dermis, a histological finding that gives the condition its name and provides crucial insights into its nature.

As we delve into the pages of this book, our goal is to provide a thorough understanding of JLI, from its microscopic origins to its impact on patients' lives. We will explore the current state of knowledge, challenge existing paradigms, and look toward future developments in diagnosis and treatment. Whether you are a dermatologist, a general practitioner, a researcher, or a patient seeking in-depth knowledge, this book aims to be your comprehensive guide to Jessner's Lymphocytic Infiltrate.

Historical Perspective

To appreciate the current understanding of JLI, we must first look back at its discovery and the evolution of our knowledge over time. Max Jessner and Norman Kanof's original description in 1953 marked the beginning of JLI as a recognized entity. Their paper, titled "Lymphocytic infiltration of the skin," published in the AMA Archives of Dermatology and Syphilology, detailed a series of cases with distinctive clinical and histological features that set them apart from other known skin conditions.

In the decades that followed, dermatologists and researchers worldwide contributed to the growing body of knowledge about JLI. Early debates centered on whether JLI was a distinct entity or a variant of other conditions such as lupus erythematosus or polymorphous light eruption. These discussions highlighted the challenges in diagnosing and categorizing skin disorders with overlapping features.

The advent of immunohistochemistry in the 1970s and 1980s brought new insights into the cellular composition of JLI lesions. Researchers were able to identify the predominant T-cell infiltrate, shedding light on the immunological nature of the condition. This period also saw increased recognition of JLI's clinical variability, with reports of cases presenting in diverse ways and affecting different demographic groups.

As we entered the 21st century, advancements in molecular biology and genetics opened new avenues for understanding JLI. While no definitive genetic markers have been identified, studies have suggested potential hereditary factors and associations with certain HLA types. These findings have paved the way for ongoing research into the underlying mechanisms of JLI and its potential relationship to other autoimmune conditions.

Epidemiology and Prevalence

One of the challenges in understanding JLI lies in determining its true prevalence. The condition is generally considered rare, but exact figures are difficult to establish due to potential underdiagnosis and misdiagnosis. JLI can affect individuals of all races and ethnicities, though some studies suggest a higher prevalence in fair-skinned populations.

Age of onset typically ranges from young adulthood to middle age, with most cases diagnosed between the ages of 30 and 50. While early reports suggested a male predominance, more recent studies indicate that JLI affects both sexes relatively equally. This shift in understanding highlights the importance of ongoing epidemiological research and the need to challenge historical assumptions in medicine.

Geographical variations in JLI prevalence have been noted, with some regions reporting higher incidences than others. Whether these differences reflect true variations in occurrence or are influenced by factors such as awareness, diagnostic practices, or environmental influences remains a subject of investigation. As global health data collection improves, we may gain a clearer picture of JLI's worldwide distribution and any associated risk factors.

Significance in Dermatology

Jessner's Lymphocytic Infiltrate occupies a unique position in the field of dermatology. While not life-threatening, it presents several challenges that make it a significant condition worthy of study and attention. First and foremost, JLI serves as a model for understanding benign lymphocytic infiltrations of the skin. By studying JLI, researchers gain insights into the complex interactions between the immune system and the skin, which can have broader implications for other dermatological and autoimmune conditions.

From a clinical perspective, JLI's significance lies in its potential for misdiagnosis and its impact on patients' quality of life. The condition's resemblance to other dermatological disorders, such as cutaneous lupus erythematosus or lymphoma, underscores the importance of accurate diagnostic techniques and the need for dermatologists to be well-versed in distinguishing JLI from its mimics. Misdiagnosis can lead to inappropriate treatments, unnecessary patient anxiety, and delayed proper management.

For patients, the chronic and recurrent nature of JLI lesions can cause significant psychological distress. The visible nature of the condition, often affecting the face and other exposed areas, can impact self-esteem and social interactions. Understanding and addressing these psychosocial aspects are crucial components of comprehensive patient care in dermatology.

Moreover, JLI presents an opportunity to study the effectiveness of various treatment modalities in managing benign but persistent skin conditions. From topical therapies to systemic medications and light-based treatments, the management of JLI encompasses a wide range of dermatological interventions. This makes it a valuable condition for evaluating treatment efficacy and developing new therapeutic approaches.

Current Understanding and Ongoing Questions

As we stand in 2024, our understanding of Jessner's Lymphocytic Infiltrate has come a long way since its initial description. We now recognize JLI as a distinct clinicopathological entity, characterized by its unique histological features and clinical presentation. The predominance of T-lymphocytes in the dermal infiltrate has been well-established, and the benign nature of the condition is widely accepted.

However, many questions remain unanswered, driving ongoing research and clinical investigations. The exact etiology of JLI continues to elude researchers. While theories range from autoimmune mechanisms to reactions against unknown antigens, a definitive cause has yet to be identified. The role of environmental factors, such as UV radiation, in triggering or exacerbating JLI is another area of active study.

The relationship between JLI and other conditions, particularly those involving cutaneous lymphocytic infiltrates, remains a subject of debate. Some researchers propose that JLI may exist on a spectrum with conditions like cutaneous lupus erythematosus or lymphocytoma cutis. Understanding these potential connections could have implications for both diagnosis and treatment.

Treatment of JLI presents its own set of challenges and questions. While various therapies have shown efficacy in managing symptoms, there is no universally effective treatment, and relapses are common. The development of targeted therapies based on a deeper understanding of JLI's pathophysiology remains an important goal for researchers and clinicians alike.

Looking Ahead: Future Directions and Hopes

As we look to the future, several exciting avenues of research and clinical practice hold promise for advancing our understanding and management of Jessner's Lymphocytic Infiltrate. Genomic and proteomic studies may uncover genetic predispositions or molecular signatures associated with JLI, potentially leading to more personalized approaches to diagnosis and treatment.

Advancements in immunology continue to shed light on the intricate workings of the skin's immune system. This growing knowledge may help elucidate the specific immunological mechanisms underlying JLI, possibly revealing new therapeutic targets. The role of regulatory T-cells, cytokine networks, and other immune mediators in JLI pathogenesis are areas ripe for further exploration.

In the realm of diagnostics, emerging technologies such as in vivo confocal microscopy and advanced imaging techniques may offer new ways to visualize and characterize JLI lesions non-invasively. These tools could potentially aid in earlier diagnosis, monitoring of disease progression, and evaluation of treatment responses.

Therapeutically, the landscape is evolving with the introduction of novel immunomodulatory agents and targeted therapies. While many of these treatments are currently being studied for more severe dermatological conditions, their potential application in JLI represents an exciting area of investigation. Additionally, combination therapies and optimized treatment protocols may improve outcomes and reduce relapse rates.

The patient perspective in JLI management is gaining increasing recognition. Future approaches are likely to place greater emphasis on quality of life measures, patient-reported outcomes, and shared decision-making in treatment plans. This holistic approach to care acknowledges the psychological and social impacts of JLI alongside its physical manifestations.

Navigating This Book

As we embark on this comprehensive exploration of Jessner's Lymphocytic Infiltrate, this book is structured to provide a logical and thorough examination of all aspects of the condition. We begin with the foundational science, delving into the intricate relationship between the immune system and the skin. This sets the stage for a detailed discussion of JLI's pathophysiology, clinical presentation, and diagnostic approaches.

The chapters on treatment and management strategies offer practical guidance for healthcare professionals, while also exploring cutting-edge research and emerging therapies. We've dedicated significant attention to the lived experience of JLI, incorporating patient perspectives and addressing the psychological aspects of the condition.

Special populations, such as pediatric and elderly patients, are given focused consideration, recognizing the unique challenges these groups may face. We also cast our gaze to the future, examining ongoing research and potential breakthroughs on the horizon.

Throughout the book, we strive to balance scientific rigor with accessibility, making the content valuable for both medical professionals and informed patients. Case studies, illustrations, and summary boxes are used to reinforce key concepts and provide real-world context.

It is our hope that this book will serve not only as a comprehensive reference on Jessner's Lymphocytic Infiltrate but also as a catalyst for further research, improved clinical practice, and enhanced patient care. As we unravel the mysteries of JLI, we contribute to the broader understanding of cutaneous immunology and inflammatory skin disorders.

In the chapters that follow, we invite you to explore the fascinating world of Jessner's Lymphocytic Infiltrate. Whether you're seeking to expand your clinical knowledge, looking for the latest research findings, or trying to understand your own condition better, this book aims to be your definitive guide. Let us begin this journey of discovery, always keeping in mind that behind every scientific fact and clinical observation is a patient whose life is affected by this intriguing condition.

CHAPTER 1

The Immune System and Skin: A Complex Relationship

The skin, our body's largest organ, serves as more than just a protective barrier against the external environment. It is a complex, multifunctional system that plays a crucial role in immune defense, sensation, temperature regulation, and even vitamin D synthesis. To fully appreciate the intricacies of Jessner's Lymphocytic Infiltrate (JLI), we must first understand the intricate relationship between the immune system and the skin. This chapter will explore the fundamental concepts of skin immunology, setting the stage for a deeper understanding of JLI and other cutaneous immune-mediated conditions.

1.1 The Structure and Functions of the Skin

The skin is composed of three main layers: the epidermis, dermis, and hypodermis (also known as the subcutaneous layer). Each layer has distinct functions and contains various cell types that contribute to the skin's overall role in immune defense.

The epidermis, the outermost layer, is primarily composed of keratinocytes. These cells form a physical barrier and produce antimicrobial peptides, contributing to innate immunity. The epidermis also contains melanocytes, which produce melanin for photoprotection, and Langerhans cells, specialized dendritic cells that play a crucial role in antigen presentation and immune surveillance.

The dermis, lying beneath the epidermis, is a connective tissue layer rich in collagen and elastin fibers. It contains blood vessels, nerve endings, hair follicles, and various glands. The dermis is home to numerous immune cells, including dermal dendritic cells, mast cells, and lymphocytes, which are central to both innate and adaptive immune responses.

The hypodermis, the deepest layer, consists mainly of adipose tissue and serves as an energy reserve, insulator, and cushion for the skin.

1.2 Overview of the Immune System

The immune system is a complex network of cells, tissues, and organs that work together to defend the body against pathogens and other harmful substances. It can be broadly divided into two main components: innate immunity and adaptive immunity.

Innate immunity provides the first line of defense against pathogens. It includes physical barriers (like the skin), chemical barriers (such as antimicrobial peptides), and cellular components (including neutrophils, macrophages, and natural killer cells). The innate immune response is rapid but non-specific.

Adaptive immunity, on the other hand, is highly specific and develops over time. It involves T lymphocytes (T cells) and B lymphocytes (B cells), which can recognize specific antigens and mount targeted responses. Adaptive immunity also has the capacity for immunological memory, allowing for faster and more effective responses to previously encountered pathogens.

1.3 Skin Immune Surveillance

The skin's immune system, often referred to as the skin-associated lymphoid tissue (SALT), is a complex network of immune cells and molecules that work together to maintain skin health and defend against pathogens.

Key players in skin immune surveillance include:

1. Keratinocytes: Beyond their structural role, keratinocytes produce antimicrobial peptides and cytokines, contributing to innate immunity and influencing adaptive immune responses.

2. Langerhans cells: These specialized dendritic cells in the epidermis capture antigens and migrate to lymph nodes, where they present these antigens to T cells, initiating adaptive immune responses.

3. Dermal dendritic cells: Similar to Langerhans cells, these cells in the dermis are efficient antigen presenters and play a crucial role in initiating and modulating immune responses.

4. T cells: Various subsets of T cells reside in the skin, including memory T cells that can rapidly respond to previously encountered antigens.

5. Innate lymphoid cells (ILCs): These cells contribute to tissue homeostasis and provide early defense against pathogens.

6. Mast cells: Located primarily in the dermis, mast cells release inflammatory mediators and play a role in allergic responses and host defense.

The orchestrated actions of these cells, along with circulating immune cells that can be recruited to the skin, form a comprehensive surveillance system capable of responding to a wide range of challenges.

1.4 T Cells in Skin Health and Disease

T lymphocytes play a central role in adaptive immunity and are particularly important in skin immunology. Several subsets of T cells are found in the skin, each with distinct functions:

1. CD4+ T helper cells (Th cells): These cells orchestrate immune responses by producing cytokines that activate other immune cells. Different subsets of Th cells (Th1, Th2, Th17, etc.) produce distinct cytokine profiles and are associated with various skin conditions.

2. CD8+ cytotoxic T cells: These cells can directly kill infected or abnormal cells and are crucial in defending against intracellular pathogens and tumors.

3. Regulatory T cells (Tregs): These cells help maintain immune tolerance and prevent excessive immune responses that could lead to autoimmunity or inflammation.

4. Tissue-resident memory T cells (TRM): These cells reside long-term in the skin and provide rapid local immune responses to previously encountered antigens.

In the context of Jessner's Lymphocytic Infiltrate, T cells are of particular interest. The characteristic lymphocytic infiltrate in JLI primarily consists of T cells, predominantly CD4+ T cells with a smaller population of CD8+ T cells. Understanding the role of these T cells in JLI pathogenesis is an active area of research and may hold keys to improved diagnosis and treatment.

1.5 Cytokines and Chemokines in Skin Immunity

Cytokines and chemokines are small proteins that act as chemical messengers in the immune system. They play crucial roles in initiating, maintaining, and resolving immune responses in the skin.

Key cytokines in skin immunity include:

1. Interferons (IFNs): These cytokines are important in antiviral responses and can also have immunomodulatory effects.

2. Interleukins (ILs): Various interleukins have diverse roles, from promoting inflammation (e.g., IL-1, IL-6) to regulating T cell differentiation (e.g., IL-12, IL-4).

3. Tumor Necrosis Factor (TNF): This pro-inflammatory cytokine is involved in various skin inflammatory conditions.

4. Transforming Growth Factor-β (TGF-β): This cytokine has both pro-inflammatory and anti-inflammatory properties and is involved in tissue repair and fibrosis.

Chemokines, a subset of cytokines, are responsible for directing the migration of immune cells. They play a crucial role in recruiting specific immune cell populations to the skin during both homeostasis and inflammation.

In JLI, alterations in cytokine and chemokine profiles may contribute to the persistent lymphocytic infiltration and the clinical manifestations of the condition. Studying these molecular mediators provides insights into disease mechanisms and potential therapeutic targets.

1.6 The Skin Microbiome and Immunity

In recent years, there has been growing recognition of the importance of the skin microbiome in maintaining skin health and modulating immune responses. The skin microbiome refers to the diverse community of microorganisms that inhabit the skin surface and appendages.

The skin microbiome interacts with the immune system in several ways:

1. Competitive exclusion: Commensal microorganisms can prevent colo-

nization by pathogenic species.

2. Antimicrobial peptide production: Some commensal bacteria produce substances that inhibit the growth of pathogens.

3. Immune education: The presence of commensal microorganisms helps shape and maintain a balanced immune response in the skin.

4. Modulation of inflammation: Certain commensal species can influence inflammatory responses, potentially playing a role in inflammatory skin conditions.

While the role of the microbiome in JLI has not been extensively studied, alterations in the skin microbiome have been implicated in various inflammatory skin conditions. Future research may reveal whether microbial factors contribute to JLI pathogenesis or if manipulating the microbiome could offer therapeutic benefits.

1.7 Immune-Mediated Skin Diseases: A Spectrum of Disorders

Understanding the complex interplay between the immune system and the skin provides a framework for comprehending a wide range of immune-mediated skin diseases. These conditions can be broadly categorized based on the predominant immune mechanisms involved:

1. T cell-mediated disorders: These include conditions like psoriasis, lichen planus, and certain forms of dermatitis. JLI falls into this category, characterized by a predominant T cell infiltrate.

2. B cell-mediated disorders: Conditions such as pemphigus and bullous pemphigoid involve autoantibodies produced by B cells.

3. Mixed immune-mediated disorders: Some conditions, like lupus erythe-

matosus, involve complex interactions between various immune cell types and mechanisms.

4. Innate immune-driven disorders: Conditions like rosacea and hidradenitis suppurativa are thought to involve dysregulation of innate immune responses.

Jessner's Lymphocytic Infiltrate, with its characteristic T cell infiltrate, shares features with other T cell-mediated skin disorders. However, its unique clinical and histological features set it apart, highlighting the complexity and diversity of immune-mediated skin conditions.

1.8 Immune Privilege in the Skin

Certain sites in the body, including parts of the skin, exhibit a phenomenon known as immune privilege. This refers to a state of reduced immune reactivity that helps protect vital structures from potentially damaging inflammatory responses.

In the skin, areas of immune privilege include:

1. Hair follicles: The lower portion of the hair follicle exhibits features of immune privilege, which is thought to play a role in hair growth cycles and may be relevant in certain forms of alopecia.

2. Sebaceous glands: These glands also show some features of immune privilege, which may help regulate local immune responses.

Understanding immune privilege in the skin provides insights into how the immune system is regulated in different skin compartments and may have implications for understanding and treating various skin conditions, potentially including JLI.

1.9 Neuroimmunology of the Skin

The skin is richly innervated, and there is growing recognition of the bidirectional communication between the nervous system and the immune system in the skin. This field, known as cutaneous neuroimmunology, explores how neural factors influence immune responses and vice versa.

Key aspects of cutaneous neuroimmunology include:

1. Neuropeptides: Substances like substance P and calcitonin gene-related peptide (CGRP) released by nerve endings can modulate immune cell function and inflammation.

2. Stress responses: Psychological stress can influence skin immune responses through neuroendocrine pathways.

3. Itch and inflammation: The interplay between itch sensations, scratch responses, and skin inflammation involves complex neuroimmune interactions.

While the role of neuroimmune interactions in JLI is not well-established, this area represents a frontier in skin immunology research that may yield new insights into various skin conditions.

1.10 Immunological Techniques in Dermatology

Advances in immunological techniques have revolutionized our understanding of skin biology and pathology. Several key methods are employed in both research and clinical practice:

1. Immunohistochemistry: This technique allows for the visualization of specific proteins or cell types in skin tissue sections, crucial for diagnosing and studying conditions like JLI.

2. Flow cytometry: This method enables the quantification and characterization of different immune cell populations in skin samples or blood.

3. Cytokine profiling: Techniques like ELISA or multiplex assays allow for the measurement of multiple cytokines, providing insights into the immune environment in various skin conditions.

4. Single-cell RNA sequencing: This cutting-edge technique provides detailed information about gene expression at the individual cell level, offering unprecedented insights into cellular heterogeneity and function in skin immunity.

5. In vivo imaging: Advanced imaging techniques like in vivo confocal microscopy allow for non-invasive visualization of skin structures and can be used to monitor immune cell dynamics in living skin.

These techniques, among others, have been instrumental in advancing our understanding of skin immunology and continue to drive progress in both basic research and clinical dermatology.

Conclusion

The relationship between the immune system and the skin is intricate, dynamic, and essential for maintaining skin health and defending against pathogens. From the physical barrier of the epidermis to the complex network of immune cells in the dermis, every aspect of skin biology is intertwined with immunological processes.

Understanding this relationship provides a crucial foundation for exploring specific skin conditions like Jessner's Lymphocytic Infiltrate. The predominance of T cells in JLI lesions, for instance, can be better appreciated in the context of normal T cell functions in the skin and their roles in other T cell-mediated skin disorders.

As we delve deeper into the specifics of JLI in subsequent chapters, we will frequently revisit these fundamental concepts of skin immunology. The complex interplay of immune cells, cytokines, and tissue-specific factors that we've explored here underlies many of the clinical and pathological features of JLI.

Moreover, this understanding of skin immunology informs current treatment approaches and guides future research directions. From topical immunomodulators to systemic therapies targeting specific immune pathways, the management of JLI and many other skin conditions is deeply rooted in immunological principles.

As our knowledge of skin immunology continues to expand, driven by advances in research techniques and clinical observations, we can anticipate new insights into conditions like JLI. These insights promise to enhance our diagnostic capabilities, refine our treatment strategies, and ultimately improve outcomes for patients affected by immune-mediated skin disorders.

In the next chapter, we will build upon this foundation to explore the specific pathophysiology of Jessner's Lymphocytic Infiltrate, examining how perturbations in normal skin immune function may contribute to the development of this intriguing condition.

CHAPTER 2

Pathophysiology of Jessner's Lymphocytic Infiltrate

Building upon our understanding of skin immunology, we now turn our attention to the specific pathophysiological mechanisms underlying Jessner's Lymphocytic Infiltrate (JLI). While the exact etiology of JLI remains elusive, decades of research have provided valuable insights into the cellular and molecular processes involved in this condition. This chapter will explore the current understanding of JLI pathophysiology, examining cellular mechanisms, genetic factors, and potential environmental triggers.

2.1 Cellular Mechanisms

The hallmark of JLI is a dense, lymphocyte-rich infiltrate in the dermis. Understanding the nature of this infiltrate and the roles of various cell types involved is crucial to unraveling the pathophysiology of the condition.

2.1.1 T Cell Predominance

Histopathological studies consistently show that the lymphocytic infiltrate in JLI is predominantly composed of T cells. Immunohistochemical analyses have revealed that these T cells are primarily CD4+ helper T cells, with a smaller population of CD8+ cytotoxic T cells. This T cell predominance suggests that JLI is primarily a T cell-mediated condition.

The specific subsets of CD4+ T cells involved in JLI have been a subject of investigation. Some studies have reported a predominance of Th1 cells, characterized by the production of interferon-γ (IFN-γ) and tumor necrosis factor-α (TNF-α). These cytokines are known to promote inflammation and may contribute to the persistent nature of JLI lesions.

Other research has identified populations of Th17 cells in JLI lesions. Th17 cells, which produce interleukin-17 (IL-17) and other pro-inflammatory cytokines, have been implicated in various autoimmune and inflammatory skin conditions. Their presence in JLI suggests a potential role in driving the inflammatory process.

The balance between effector T cells and regulatory T cells (Tregs) is crucial for maintaining immune homeostasis. Some studies have reported a relative decrease in Tregs in JLI lesions, which could contribute to the persistent inflammation characteristic of the condition.

2.1.2 Role of Antigen-Presenting Cells

While T cells form the bulk of the cellular infiltrate in JLI, antigen-presenting cells (APCs) play a crucial role in initiating and sustaining the immune response. Dendritic cells, including both Langerhans cells from the epidermis and dermal dendritic cells, have been observed in increased numbers in JLI lesions.

These APCs are thought to present as-yet-unidentified antigens to T cells, triggering their activation and proliferation. The nature of these putative antigens – whether they are self-antigens, environmental antigens, or microbial components – remains a subject of ongoing research and debate.

2.1.3 Other Cellular Components

While less prominent than T cells, other cell types contribute to the pathophysiology of JLI:

1. B cells: Although not a major component of the infiltrate, small numbers of B cells have been observed in some JLI lesions. Their exact role in the condition is not well understood.

2. Macrophages: These cells are present in the infiltrate and may contribute to inflammation through cytokine production and phagocytosis.

3. Mast cells: Some studies have reported increased numbers of mast cells in JLI lesions. These cells can release various inflammatory mediators and may contribute to the pathogenesis of the condition.

4. Keratinocytes: While not part of the infiltrate, keratinocytes in JLI lesions show signs of activation, including increased expression of intercellular adhesion molecule-1 (ICAM-1). This may facilitate the recruitment and retention of immune cells in the skin.

2.2 Molecular Mechanisms

The cellular interactions in JLI are mediated by a complex network of molecular signals, including cytokines, chemokines, and adhesion molecules.

2.2.1 Cytokine Profile

Analysis of cytokine expression in JLI lesions has provided insights into the inflammatory milieu driving the condition. Key findings include:

1. Elevated levels of IFN-γ and TNF-α, consistent with a Th1-type immune response.
2. Increased expression of IL-17 and IL-22, suggesting involvement of the Th17 pathway.

3. Presence of IL-2, a cytokine crucial for T cell proliferation and survival.
4. Variability in levels of immunoregulatory cytokines like IL-10 and TGF-β, which may reflect attempts to modulate the inflammatory response.

The cytokine profile in JLI shares similarities with other T cell-mediated skin conditions but also exhibits unique features that may account for its distinctive clinical presentation.

2.2.2 Chemokines and Cell Trafficking

The recruitment and retention of lymphocytes in JLI lesions involve various chemokines and adhesion molecules. Studies have identified increased expression of:

1. CXCL9, CXCL10, and CXCL11: These chemokines attract CXCR3-expressing T cells, which are predominantly of the Th1 type.
2. CCL17 and CCL22: These chemokines bind to CCR4, which is expressed on various T cell subsets, including skin-homing T cells.
3. Adhesion molecules: Upregulation of molecules like ICAM-1 on keratinocytes and vascular endothelium facilitates lymphocyte adhesion and migration into the skin.

The specific pattern of chemokine expression in JLI may help explain the localized nature of the lesions and the predominance of certain T cell subsets in the infiltrate.

2.2.3 Apoptosis and Cell Turnover

The persistence of JLI lesions suggests a dysregulation in the normal processes of cell turnover and resolution of inflammation. Some studies have investigated the role of apoptosis in JLI:

1. Altered expression of apoptosis-related proteins: Changes in the balance between pro-apoptotic (e.g., Bax) and anti-apoptotic (e.g., Bcl-2) proteins may contribute to the accumulation of lymphocytes in JLI lesions.
2. Fas/Fas ligand system: This pathway, important for the regulation of T cell homeostasis, has been found to be altered in some cases of JLI.

Understanding these mechanisms may provide insights into why the lymphocytic infiltrate in JLI persists and potential therapeutic approaches to promote its resolution.

2.3 Genetic Factors

While JLI is not typically considered a hereditary condition, genetic factors may play a role in susceptibility to the disorder and influence its clinical presentation.

2.3.1 HLA Associations

Several studies have investigated potential associations between JLI and human leukocyte antigen (HLA) types. Some findings include:

1. Increased frequency of HLA-B8 and HLA-DR3 in some JLI patient populations.
2. Associations with HLA-DQA1*0501 in certain ethnic groups.

These HLA associations, while not consistent across all studies, suggest that genetic factors influencing antigen presentation may contribute to JLI susceptibility.

2.3.2 Familial Cases

Although rare, familial cases of JLI have been reported in the literature. These cases provide compelling evidence for a genetic component in at least some instances of the condition. Analyses of familial cases have suggested:

1. Possible autosomal dominant inheritance pattern in some families.
2. Variable penetrance and expressivity, indicating the likely influence of additional genetic or environmental factors.

2.3.3 Genetic Polymorphisms

Research into genetic polymorphisms associated with JLI is still in its early stages, but some studies have explored:

1. Cytokine gene polymorphisms: Variations in genes encoding cytokines like TNF-α and IL-10 have been investigated for potential associations with JLI.
2. T cell receptor gene rearrangements: Some studies have examined T cell receptor gene rearrangements in JLI lesions, looking for evidence of clonal T cell expansion.

While these genetic studies have not yet yielded definitive results, they represent an important avenue for future research that may enhance our understanding of JLI pathogenesis and individual susceptibility.

2.4 Environmental Triggers

The role of environmental factors in triggering or exacerbating JLI has been a subject of ongoing investigation. Several potential triggers have been proposed:

2.4.1 Ultraviolet Radiation

UV radiation has been implicated as a potential trigger or exacerbating factor in JLI:

1. Photosensitivity: Some patients with JLI report worsening of lesions with sun exposure.
2. Seasonal variation: Cases of JLI have been observed to fluctuate with seasons in some patients, with increased incidence or severity during summer months.
3. UV-induced immunomodulation: UV radiation is known to have complex effects on skin immunity, which may contribute to the pathogenesis of JLI in susceptible individuals.

However, it's important to note that not all patients with JLI demonstrate photosensitivity, and the role of UV radiation may vary among individuals.

2.4.2 Infectious Agents

The possibility of infectious triggers for JLI has been explored, although no consistent associations have been established:

1. Borrelia burgdorferi: Some studies have investigated a potential link between JLI and Borrelia infection, but results have been inconsistent

across different geographic regions.

2. Viral infections: Cases of JLI-like eruptions following viral infections have been reported, suggesting a possible role for viral triggers in some instances.

The inconsistent findings regarding infectious triggers highlight the likely multifactorial nature of JLI and the possibility that different environmental factors may be relevant in different patient subgroups.

2.4.3 Medications and Chemical Exposures

Various medications and chemical exposures have been reported as potential triggers for JLI-like eruptions:

1. Drug-induced cases: Reports of JLI-like reactions following administration of certain medications, including anticonvulsants and antihypertensives, suggest that drug hypersensitivity may mimic or trigger JLI in some cases.
2. Occupational exposures: Some case reports have linked JLI to occupational exposures to various chemicals, although these associations remain anecdotal.

These observations underscore the importance of thorough history-taking in patients presenting with JLI-like lesions to identify potential environmental triggers.

2.5 Immunological Dysfunction Hypotheses

Several hypotheses have been proposed to explain the underlying immunological dysfunction in JLI:

2.5.1 Autoimmune Hypothesis

Some researchers have suggested that JLI may represent a form of autoimmune response directed against skin components:

1. Loss of self-tolerance: The persistent T cell infiltrate may reflect a breakdown in immunological tolerance to skin antigens.
2. Molecular mimicry: It's been hypothesized that environmental antigens (e.g., from infectious agents) may share similarities with skin components, leading to cross-reactive immune responses.

However, the lack of systemic symptoms or progression to more generalized autoimmune conditions in most JLI patients has led some to question the autoimmune hypothesis.

2.5.2 Delayed-Type Hypersensitivity Reaction

Another perspective views JLI as a form of delayed-type hypersensitivity reaction to an unknown antigen:

1. Persistent antigen presence: The chronic nature of JLI lesions may reflect ongoing exposure to an environmental antigen or retention of antigen in the skin.
2. T cell memory: The predominance of memory T cells in JLI infiltrates supports the idea of an ongoing response to a specific antigen.

This hypothesis aligns with the T cell-dominated histology of JLI but leaves open the question of the nature and source of the putative antigen.

2.5.3 Dysregulated Immune Response Hypothesis

Some researchers propose that JLI represents a more fundamental dysregulation of skin immune responses:

1. Impaired resolution of inflammation: The persistent nature of JLI lesions may reflect a failure of normal mechanisms for resolving skin inflammation.
2. Altered T cell homeostasis: Imbalances in T cell subsets, particularly between effector and regulatory T cells, may contribute to ongoing inflammation.

This perspective views JLI as a model of dysregulated skin immunity that may have relevance to understanding other chronic inflammatory skin conditions.

2.6 Integrating Pathophysiological Insights

As we synthesize the various aspects of JLI pathophysiology, several key points emerge:

1. T cell centrality: The predominance of T cells, particularly CD4+ T cells, in JLI lesions underscores the central role of these cells in the condition's pathogenesis.

2. Cytokine-mediated inflammation: The specific cytokine profile in JLI lesions, characterized by elevated levels of Th1 and Th17-associated cytokines, drives the inflammatory process and shapes the clinical presentation.

3. Multifactorial etiology: The interplay of genetic susceptibility factors and environmental triggers likely contributes to the development of JLI, explain-

ing its sporadic occurrence and variable presentation among individuals.

4. Persistent immune activation: The chronic nature of JLI lesions reflects ongoing immune activation, possibly due to persistent antigen presence, impaired regulatory mechanisms, or both.

5. Localized immune dysfunction: The localized nature of JLI lesions suggests that the underlying immune dysfunction is specific to the skin microenvironment rather than a systemic immune disorder.

Understanding these pathophysiological aspects of JLI not only enhances our comprehension of the condition but also informs diagnostic approaches and treatment strategies. The predominance of T cells and the specific cytokine profile in JLI lesions, for instance, guide the use of immunohisto-chemical staining in diagnosis and suggest potential targets for therapeutic interventions.

Moreover, recognizing the potential role of environmental triggers in JLI can inform patient management strategies, including recommendations for sun protection and the importance of identifying and avoiding potential exacerbating factors.

Conclusion

The pathophysiology of Jessner's Lymphocytic Infiltrate is complex and multifaceted, involving intricate interactions between various immune cells, molecular mediators, genetic factors, and environmental influences. While significant progress has been made in understanding the cellular and molecular aspects of JLI, many questions remain unanswered.

Future research directions may include:

1. More detailed characterization of the T cell subsets involved in JLI using advanced techniques like single-cell RNA sequencing.
2. Identification of potential autoantigens or environmental antigens that may trigger the condition.
3. Further exploration of genetic susceptibility factors through genome-wide association studies.
4. Investigation of the role of the skin microbiome in JLI pathogenesis.
5. Development of animal models to study JLI mechanisms and test potential therapeutic approaches.

As our understanding of JLI pathophysiology continues to evolve, it promises to yield new insights that will enhance diagnosis, guide the development of targeted therapies, and ultimately improve outcomes for patients with this intriguing condition. In the following chapters, we will explore how these pathophysiological insights translate into clinical presentation, diagnostic approaches, and treatment strategies for Jessner's Lymphocytic Infiltrate.

CHAPTER 3

Clinical Presentation and Symptoms of Jessner's Lymphocytic Infiltrate

Building upon our understanding of the pathophysiology of Jessner's Lymphocytic Infiltrate (JLI), we now turn our attention to its clinical manifestations. The way JLI presents clinically is crucial for diagnosis, management, and distinguishing it from other similar conditions. This chapter will explore the typical and atypical presentations of JLI, its distribution patterns, associated symptoms, and the patient experience.

3.1 Typical Lesion Characteristics

JLI is characterized by distinctive cutaneous lesions that, while variable, share common features across most patients.

3.1.1 Morphology

The primary lesions of JLI typically present as:

1. Papules: Small, raised lesions usually measuring 2-10 mm in diameter.
2. Plaques: Larger, flattened lesions that may result from the coalescence of papules.

These lesions are typically well-demarcated with a smooth surface. They are usually described as:

- Erythematous: The lesions have a reddish appearance due to increased blood flow and inflammation.
    - Non-scaly: Unlike some other inflammatory skin conditions, JLI lesions typically lack surface scaling.
    - Firm: On palpation, the lesions feel firm due to the dense dermal infiltrate.

In some cases, a subtle central depression may be observed, giving the lesions a somewhat annular appearance.

3.1.2 Color

The color of JLI lesions can vary, but they are most commonly described as:

- Pink to red: In fair-skinned individuals, lesions often appear bright red.
    - Violaceous: Some lesions may take on a purplish hue, especially in more longstanding cases.
    - Hyperpigmented: In darker-skinned individuals, lesions may appear as hyperpigmented patches or plaques.

It's important to note that the color can change over time and may be influenced by factors such as sun exposure or treatment.

3.1.3 Evolution of Lesions

JLI lesions typically follow a characteristic evolution:

1. Onset: Lesions usually appear suddenly, often developing over a few days to weeks.

2. Progression: Individual lesions may enlarge slowly over time, and new lesions may continue to appear.
3. Persistence: Without treatment, lesions can persist for months to years.
4. Resolution: Spontaneous resolution can occur, often leaving no scarring, although post-inflammatory hyperpigmentation may be observed, especially in darker skin types.

3.2 Distribution Patterns

The distribution of JLI lesions is an important aspect of its clinical presentation and can aid in diagnosis.

3.2.1 Common Sites

JLI has a predilection for certain areas of the body:

1. Face: The cheeks, forehead, and nose are commonly affected areas.
2. Neck: Both the anterior and posterior aspects of the neck may be involved.
3. Upper back: This is another frequently affected site.
4. Chest: Lesions on the upper chest are not uncommon.

3.2.2 Less Common Sites

While less frequent, JLI can occur in other areas:

1. Arms and shoulders
2. Scalp
3. Lower back

4. Rarely, other parts of the body

3.2.3 Distribution Patterns

Several distribution patterns have been observed in JLI:

1. Localized: Some patients present with a single cluster of lesions in one area.
2. Asymmetrical: It's common for lesions to be asymmetrically distributed.
3. Multifocal: Multiple discrete areas may be affected simultaneously.
4. Generalized: In rare cases, a more widespread distribution has been reported.

3.2.4 Mucosal Involvement

JLI typically does not involve mucous membranes. The absence of mucosal lesions can be a helpful distinguishing feature from some other conditions that may mimic JLI.

3.3 Associated Symptoms

While JLI is often described as an asymptomatic condition, a range of associated symptoms have been reported by patients.

3.3.1 Cutaneous Symptoms

1. Pruritus (itching): While classically described as non-pruritic, a significant proportion of patients report some degree of itching associated with their lesions.

2. Burning or tingling sensations: Some patients describe a burning or tingling feeling in affected areas.
3. Tenderness: Lesions may be tender to touch in some cases.

The intensity of these symptoms can vary widely among patients and may fluctuate over time.

3.3.2 Photosensitivity

A subset of patients with JLI report photosensitivity:

1. Exacerbation with sun exposure: Some patients notice worsening of existing lesions or development of new lesions following sun exposure.
2. Photoaggravated symptoms: Symptoms like itching or burning may increase with sun exposure in photosensitive individuals.

However, it's important to note that not all patients with JLI experience photosensitivity, and the role of UV radiation in JLI remains a subject of ongoing research.

3.3.3 Systemic Symptoms

JLI is primarily a cutaneous condition, and systemic symptoms are not typically a feature. However, some patients report:

1. Fatigue: A general sense of tiredness has been noted by some patients, although it's unclear if this is directly related to JLI or secondary to the psychological impact of the condition.
2. Mild malaise: Some patients describe a vague sense of unwellness,

particularly during flares of the condition.

The absence of significant systemic symptoms is an important feature that helps distinguish JLI from some systemic autoimmune conditions that may have similar cutaneous manifestations.

3.4 Variations in Clinical Presentation

While the classic presentation of JLI is well-described, variations and atypical presentations have been reported in the literature.

3.4.1 Morphological Variants

1. Reticular JLI: In this variant, lesions may have a net-like or reticulated appearance.
2. Annular JLI: Lesions with a ring-like configuration have been described in some cases.
3. Linear JLI: Rarely, lesions may follow a linear distribution, possibly corresponding to Blaschko's lines.

3.4.2 Pigmentary Changes

1. Hypopigmented JLI: In some cases, particularly in darker-skinned individuals, JLI lesions may present as hypopigmented rather than erythematous areas.
2. Poikilodermatous JLI: A combination of hyperpigmentation, hypopigmentation, and telangiectasias has been reported in rare cases.

3.4.3 Age-related Variations

While JLI typically affects adults, cases have been reported across the age spectrum:

1. Pediatric JLI: Cases in children and adolescents have been described, often with similar clinical features to adult cases.
2. Geriatric JLI: Older adults may present with JLI, sometimes with more subtle clinical findings due to age-related changes in the skin.

3.4.4 Extent of Involvement

The extent of skin involvement in JLI can vary widely:

1. Localized JLI: Some patients present with only a few lesions confined to a small area.
2. Extensive JLI: Rarely, patients may present with widespread lesions covering large areas of the body.

Understanding these variations in clinical presentation is crucial for accurate diagnosis and appropriate management of JLI.

3.5 Temporal Patterns and Course of Disease

The natural history of JLI can vary significantly among patients, but certain patterns have been observed.

3.5.1 Onset

1. Acute onset: Many patients report a sudden appearance of lesions over days to weeks.
2. Gradual onset: In some cases, lesions may develop more slowly over months.

3.5.2 Disease Course

JLI typically follows a chronic course with several possible patterns:

1. Persistent: Lesions may persist unchanged for months to years.
2. Relapsing-remitting: Some patients experience periods of improvement followed by recurrences.
3. Gradually progressive: In some cases, the number or extent of lesions may increase over time.
4. Spontaneous resolution: A subset of patients experience spontaneous clearance of lesions, although recurrence is possible.

3.5.3 Seasonal Variations

Some patients report seasonal fluctuations in their condition:

1. Summer exacerbations: In photosensitive individuals, lesions may worsen during summer months.
2. Winter improvement: Some patients note improvement in colder months, possibly due to reduced sun exposure.

However, these patterns are not universal, and many patients do not experience significant seasonal variations.

3.6 Factors Influencing Clinical Presentation

Several factors can influence the clinical presentation of JLI:

3.6.1 Skin Type

The appearance of JLI lesions can vary depending on the patient's skin type:

1. Fair skin: Lesions typically appear more erythematous.
2. Dark skin: Lesions may be more subtle, appearing as hyperpigmented or sometimes hypopigmented areas.

3.6.2 Age

The age of the patient can affect the clinical presentation:

1. Younger patients: May have more pronounced erythema and potentially more symptomatic lesions.
2. Older patients: May have more subtle presentations due to age-related changes in skin vascularity and immune responses.

3.6.3 Duration of Disease

The appearance of lesions may change over time:

1. Early lesions: Often more erythematous and potentially more symptomatic.
2. Chronic lesions: May become less inflamed in appearance but more

persistent.

3.6.4 Environmental Factors

Various environmental factors can influence the presentation:

1. Sun exposure: Can exacerbate lesions in photosensitive individuals.
2. Climate: Humidity and temperature may affect symptom severity in some patients.
3. Occupational exposures: Certain chemicals or irritants may influence the appearance or symptoms of JLI lesions.

3.7 Impact on Quality of Life

While JLI is not life-threatening, it can significantly impact a patient's quality of life.

3.7.1 Psychological Impact

The visible nature of JLI lesions, particularly when they occur on the face, can lead to:

1. Decreased self-esteem
2. Social anxiety
3. Depression in some cases

3.7.2 Functional Impairment

Although JLI does not typically cause significant physical impairment, patients may experience:

1. Discomfort from symptomatic lesions
2. Limitations in activities due to photosensitivity
3. Sleep disturbances if lesions are pruritic

3.7.3 Social and Occupational Effects

JLI can impact various aspects of a patient's life:

1. Social interactions: Visible lesions may lead to self-consciousness in social situations.
2. Occupational challenges: Particularly in professions requiring public interaction or sun exposure.
3. Relationship issues: Some patients report that their condition affects intimate relationships.

Understanding these quality of life impacts is crucial for comprehensive patient care and may influence treatment decisions.

3.8 Clinical Presentation in Special Populations

3.8.1 Pediatric Patients

While less common, JLI can occur in children and adolescents:

1. Clinical features are generally similar to adult cases.

2. Differential diagnosis may be broader, including conditions more common in younger age groups.
3. Psychological impact may be particularly significant during formative years.

3.8.2 Pregnancy

JLI during pregnancy presents unique considerations:

1. Hormonal influences may affect disease activity.
2. Treatment options may be limited due to safety concerns.
3. Post-partum course can be variable, with some patients experiencing improvement and others worsening.

3.8.3 Immunocompromised Patients

In immunocompromised individuals, JLI may present atypically:

1. Lesions may be more extensive or persistent.
2. Differential diagnosis becomes more complex, requiring careful exclusion of infectious or neoplastic processes.

3.9 Patient-Reported Experiences

Understanding the patient perspective is crucial for comprehensive care. Common themes in patient-reported experiences include:

1. Frustration with the chronic and unpredictable nature of the condition.
2. Anxiety about the visibility of lesions, particularly on the face.
3. Confusion due to the rarity of the condition and sometimes conflicting information.
4. Relief when receiving a definitive diagnosis, often after a period of uncertainty.
5. Varied experiences with treatments, highlighting the need for individualized management approaches.

3.10 Clinical Evaluation and Documentation

Thorough clinical evaluation and documentation are essential for diagnosis, management, and monitoring of JLI:

3.10.1 History Taking

Key elements of the patient history include:

1. Onset and evolution of lesions
2. Associated symptoms
3. Exacerbating or alleviating factors
4. Previous treatments and responses
5. Impact on quality of life

3.10.2 Physical Examination

A comprehensive skin examination should include:

1. Detailed description of lesion morphology, color, and distribution

2. Assessment of involved and uninvolved skin
3. Examination of mucous membranes and nail beds
4. Lymph node palpation

3.10.3 Photography

Clinical photography can be valuable for:

1. Documenting the initial presentation
2. Monitoring disease progression or treatment response
3. Facilitating comparison over time

3.10.4 Scoring Systems

While no standardized scoring system exists specifically for JLI, adapting scales used for other inflammatory skin conditions may be helpful for monitoring disease activity and treatment response.

Conclusion

The clinical presentation of Jessner's Lymphocytic Infiltrate is characterized by its distinctive cutaneous lesions, typically erythematous papules or plaques with a predilection for the face, neck, and upper trunk. While often described as asymptomatic, many patients experience associated symptoms such as pruritus or photosensitivity. The chronic and sometimes unpredictable course of JLI can significantly impact a patient's quality of life.

Understanding the range of clinical presentations, including typical features and variations, is crucial for accurate diagnosis and effective management of JLI. The absence of systemic symptoms, the characteristic distribution of lesions, and the histopathological findings (which will be discussed in the next chapter) help distinguish JLI from other conditions with similar cutaneous manifestations.

As we move forward, this understanding of the clinical presentation will inform our approach to diagnosis, differential diagnosis, and treatment strategies for Jessner's Lymphocytic Infiltrate. In the next chapter, we will explore the diagnostic techniques and procedures used to confirm JLI and exclude other conditions.

CHAPTER 4

D iagnostic Techniques and Procedures for Jessner's Lymphocytic Infiltrate

Accurate diagnosis of Jessner's Lymphocytic Infiltrate (JLI) is crucial for appropriate management and differentiation from other similar conditions. This chapter will explore the various diagnostic techniques and procedures used to confirm JLI, with a focus on histopathological findings, immunohistochemistry, and other advanced diagnostic tools.

4.1 Clinical Diagnosis

While laboratory investigations and histopathology are essential for confirming JLI, the initial diagnosis often begins with clinical assessment.

4.1.1 Key Clinical Features

Clinicians should be alert to the following features suggestive of JLI:

1. Erythematous papules or plaques, typically non-scaly
2. Predilection for face, neck, and upper trunk
3. Absence of significant systemic symptoms
4. Chronic or relapsing-remitting course

4.1.2 Importance of Thorough History and Examination

A comprehensive history and physical examination are crucial:

1. Onset and evolution of lesions
2. Associated symptoms, including photosensitivity
3. Previous treatments and responses
4. Complete skin examination, including mucous membranes
5. Assessment of lymph nodes

4.1.3 Clinical Photography

Standardized clinical photography can be valuable for:

1. Documenting the initial presentation
2. Monitoring disease progression
3. Evaluating treatment response over time

4.2 Skin Biopsy: The Gold Standard

Skin biopsy remains the gold standard for diagnosing JLI. The choice of biopsy technique and site is crucial for obtaining diagnostic results.

4.2.1 Biopsy Techniques

Several biopsy techniques may be employed:

1. Punch biopsy: Most commonly used, typically 4-6mm in diameter
   - Advantages: Provides full-thickness sample, relatively simple to perform

- Disadvantages: Limited sample size, may require sutures

2. Incisional biopsy: Used for larger lesions or when a larger sample is needed
   - Advantages: Larger sample size, can include normal surrounding skin
   - Disadvantages: More invasive, requires sutures, potential for scarring

3. Shave biopsy: Generally not preferred for JLI diagnosis
   - Advantages: Quick, no sutures required
   - Disadvantages: May not provide adequate depth for full assessment

4.2.2 Biopsy Site Selection

Choosing the appropriate biopsy site is crucial:

1. Select a well-developed, representative lesion
2. Avoid heavily sun-damaged areas if possible
3. Consider cosmetic implications, especially on the face
4. Include some normal-appearing skin at the edge of the lesion if possible

4.2.3 Multiple Biopsies

In some cases, multiple biopsies may be necessary:

1. When lesions have varying appearances
2. To evaluate disease progression over time
3. To assess treatment response

4.3 Histopathological Findings

The histopathological features of JLI are distinctive and form the cornerstone of diagnosis.

4.3.1 Key Histological Features

1. Dense lymphocytic infiltrate: The hallmark of JLI is a dense, sleeve-like lymphocytic infiltrate in the papillary and upper reticular dermis.

2. Perivascular and periadnexal distribution: The infiltrate typically shows a perivascular and periadnexal pattern.

3. Epidermal changes: The epidermis is usually normal or may show slight acanthosis. Typically, there is no significant interface change.

4. Mucin deposition: Increased dermal mucin may be observed, although this is not a consistent feature.

5. Absence of other significant changes: There is typically no significant fibrosis, no follicular plugging, and no atrophy of the epidermis.

4.3.2 Cellular Composition of the Infiltrate

1. Predominance of T lymphocytes: The majority of cells in the infiltrate are T lymphocytes.

2. Mixture of cell types: While T cells predominate, other cell types may be present in smaller numbers, including B cells, plasma cells, and histiocytes.

3. Absence of atypical cells: The lymphocytes appear mature and well-differentiated, without significant atypia.

4.3.3 Special Stains

Several special stains may be employed to enhance the histological diagnosis:

1. Giemsa or toluidine blue: To identify mast cells
2. Alcian blue: To highlight dermal mucin deposition
3. Elastic van Gieson: To assess for changes in dermal elastic fibers

4.4 Immunohistochemistry

Immunohistochemical staining plays a crucial role in characterizing the cellular infiltrate in JLI and differentiating it from other conditions.

4.4.1 T Cell Markers

1. CD3: Pan-T cell marker, positive in the majority of infiltrating cells
2. CD4: Helper T cell marker, typically predominant
3. CD8: Cytotoxic T cell marker, present but usually in smaller numbers

4.4.2 B Cell Markers

1. CD20: B cell marker, may be positive in a small proportion of cells

4.4.3 Other Relevant Markers

1. CD68: Macrophage marker
2. S100: Dendritic cell marker
3. Ki-67: Proliferation marker, usually low in JLI

4.4.4 Interpretation of Immunohistochemistry Results

1. T cell predominance: Confirms the T cell-rich nature of the infiltrate
2. CD4:CD8 ratio: Typically shows CD4 predominance
3. Low Ki-67 index: Indicates a low proliferative rate, helping to distinguish from cutaneous lymphomas

4.5 Molecular Diagnostic Techniques

While not routinely required for diagnosis, molecular techniques can provide additional information in challenging cases.

4.5.1 T Cell Receptor Gene Rearrangement Studies

1. Purpose: To assess for clonality of the T cell infiltrate
2. Technique: PCR-based analysis of T cell receptor genes
3. Interpretation: Polyclonal results support a benign, reactive process like JLI, while monoclonal results may suggest a T cell lymphoma

4.5.2 In Situ Hybridization

1. EBER (Epstein-Barr virus-encoded RNA) in situ hybridization: To exclude EBV-associated lymphoproliferative disorders

4.5.3 Next-Generation Sequencing

While not currently part of routine diagnosis, next-generation sequencing techniques may offer future insights into the genetic basis of JLI and help in difficult-to-diagnose cases.

4.6 Laboratory Investigations

While JLI is primarily a clinical and histopathological diagnosis, laboratory tests can help exclude other conditions and assess for associated abnormalities.

4.6.1 Routine Blood Tests

1. Complete blood count (CBC): Usually normal in JLI
2. Erythrocyte sedimentation rate (ESR) and C-reactive protein (CRP): Typically normal, elevated levels may suggest alternative diagnoses

4.6.2 Autoimmune Serologies

To help exclude systemic autoimmune conditions:

1. Antinuclear antibodies (ANA)
2. Extractable nuclear antigens (ENA)
3. Anti-double-stranded DNA antibodies

4.6.3 Other Relevant Tests

Depending on the clinical presentation and suspected differential diagnoses:

1. Serum protein electrophoresis: To exclude paraproteinemias
2. Borrelia serology: In cases where Borrelia infection is suspected
3. Hepatitis B and C serology: To exclude virus-associated lesions

4.7 Imaging Studies

Imaging studies are not routinely required for diagnosing JLI but may be helpful in certain situations.

4.7.1 Dermoscopy

While not diagnostic, dermoscopy can provide additional information:

1. Characteristic features: Unfocused vessels, whitish structureless areas
2. Utility: Can help guide biopsy site selection and monitor treatment response

4.7.2 Reflectance Confocal Microscopy (RCM)

An emerging non-invasive imaging technique:

1. Allows visualization of cellular details in vivo
2. Can show characteristic features of JLI, including the dense lymphocytic infiltrate
3. Potential for monitoring disease activity and treatment response without repeated biopsies

4.7.3 Other Imaging Modalities

Rarely, other imaging studies may be employed:

1. Ultrasonography: To assess depth and extent of lesions in atypical cases

2. CT or MRI: Generally not indicated unless there's suspicion of deeper involvement or to exclude other conditions

4.8 Diagnostic Criteria and Algorithms

While no universally accepted diagnostic criteria exist for JLI, several authors have proposed criteria based on a combination of clinical, histopathological, and immunohistochemical features.

4.8.1 Proposed Diagnostic Criteria

A diagnosis of JLI can be considered when the following are present:

1. Clinical features:
   - Erythematous papules or plaques
   - Predilection for face, neck, and upper trunk
   - Absence of significant systemic symptoms

2. Histopathological features:
   - Dense, perivascular and periadnexal lymphocytic infiltrate
   - Relative sparing of the epidermis
   - Absence of significant interface change or other specific features of lupus erythematosus

3. Immunohistochemical features:
   - Predominance of CD3+ T cells
   - CD4+ T cells outnumbering CD8+ T cells
   - Absence of monoclonal B cell populations

4. Exclusion of other similar conditions through appropriate investigations

4.8.2 Diagnostic Algorithm

A step-wise approach to diagnosing JLI might include:

1. Clinical suspicion based on characteristic lesions and distribution
2. Skin biopsy for histopathology and immunohistochemistry
3. Basic laboratory investigations to exclude systemic conditions
4. Consider additional tests (e.g., T cell receptor gene rearrangement) in equivocal cases
5. Synthesis of all findings to reach a diagnosis
6. Re-evaluation and possible repeat biopsy if the diagnosis remains unclear

4.9 Differential Diagnosis

A wide range of conditions can mimic JLI clinically or histologically, making a thorough differential diagnosis crucial.

4.9.1 Cutaneous Lupus Erythematosus (CLE)

1. Clinical similarities: Erythematous plaques, photosensitivity
2. Distinguishing features:

- CLE often shows epidermal changes and interface dermatitis histologically
    - Positive ANA and other autoantibodies in systemic lupus

4.9.2 Polymorphous Light Eruption (PMLE)

1. Clinical similarities: Photodistributed erythematous papules or plaques
2. Distinguishing features:

- PMLE is typically seasonal and resolves more quickly
  - Histology of PMLE is more variable and often less dense than JLI

4.9.3 Cutaneous Lymphoma

1. Clinical similarities: Persistent erythematous patches or plaques
2. Distinguishing features:

- Cutaneous lymphomas often show atypical lymphocytes histologically
  - T cell receptor gene rearrangement studies may show clonality in lymphomas

4.9.4 Pseudolymphoma

1. Clinical similarities: Persistent lymphocytic infiltrates
2. Distinguishing features:

- Pseudolymphomas often have a known trigger (e.g., medication, infection)
  - May show a more mixed cellular infiltrate histologically

4.9.5 Reticular Erythematous Mucinosis (REM)

1. Clinical similarities: Erythematous plaques, often on the chest
2. Distinguishing features:

- REM typically shows more prominent mucin deposition histologically
  - Often has a reticular or net-like clinical appearance

4.9.6 Lymphocytoma Cutis

1. Clinical similarities: Persistent lymphocytic infiltrates
2. Distinguishing features:

- Often presents as a solitary nodule
  - May show germinal center formation histologically

4.9.7 Sarcoidosis

1. Clinical similarities: Can present with erythematous plaques
2. Distinguishing features:

- Sarcoidosis shows characteristic granulomas histologically
  - Often associated with systemic symptoms

4.10 Challenges in Diagnosis

Despite advances in diagnostic techniques, JLI can present diagnostic challenges.

4.10.1 Overlap with Other Conditions

1. Some cases may show features overlapping with CLE or other conditions
2. The concept of "JLI-like" lesions in the setting of other disorders

4.10.2 Variability in Histological Findings

1. Depends on the stage and activity of the lesion biopsied
2. Influence of previous treatments on histological appearance

4.10.3 Limitations of Current Diagnostic Tools

1. Lack of specific biomarkers for JLI
2. Potential sampling error in biopsy

4.10.4 Evolving Understanding of the Condition

1. Ongoing debates about the exact nature and classification of JLI
2. Potential for new subtypes or related conditions to be identified

4.11 Future Directions in JLI Diagnosis

As our understanding of JLI evolves, new diagnostic approaches may emerge.

4.11.1 Advanced Imaging Techniques

1. Further development of in vivo confocal microscopy for non-invasive diagnosis
2. Potential applications of artificial intelligence in image analysis

4.11.2 Molecular Profiling

1. Gene expression profiling to identify specific signatures of JLI
2. Proteomics approaches to identify potential biomarkers

4.11.3 Microbiome Studies

1. Investigation of potential roles of skin microbiome in JLI pathogenesis
2. Microbiome profiling as a diagnostic or prognostic tool

4.11.4 Improved Classification Systems

1. Development of more refined diagnostic criteria
2. Potential for subclassification of JLI based on clinical, histological, or molecular features

Conclusion

Accurate diagnosis of Jessner's Lymphocytic Infiltrate relies on a combination of clinical assessment, histopathology, immunohistochemistry, and sometimes molecular studies. The characteristic dense, T cell-rich lymphocytic infiltrate in the dermis, coupled with the typical clinical presentation, forms the basis of diagnosis. However, the similarity to other conditions necessitates a thorough diagnostic workup and careful exclusion of mimics.

As our understanding of JLI continues to evolve, so too will our diagnostic approaches. The integration of advanced imaging techniques, molecular profiling, and potentially microbiome studies may offer new insights and improve our ability to diagnose and classify this intriguing condition accurately.

In the next chapter, we will explore the various treatment modalities available for managing Jessner's Lymphocytic Infiltrate, building upon the diagnostic framework established here.

CHAPTER 5

Treatment Modalities: Current Standards and Emerging Therapies

The management of Jessner's Lymphocytic Infiltrate (JLI) presents unique challenges due to its chronic nature, variable presentation, and the lack of a universally effective treatment. This chapter will explore the current treatment modalities available for JLI, ranging from well-established approaches to emerging therapies. We will discuss the efficacy, limitations, and considerations for each treatment option, providing a comprehensive guide for clinicians managing this condition.

5.1 Treatment Goals and Considerations

Before delving into specific treatments, it's important to establish the goals of therapy and key considerations in managing JLI.

5.1.1 Treatment Goals

1. Symptomatic relief: Alleviate associated symptoms such as pruritus or burning sensations
2. Cosmetic improvement: Reduce the visibility of lesions, particularly on exposed areas
3. Disease control: Prevent the development of new lesions and control existing ones

4. Quality of life enhancement: Improve the patient's overall well-being and functional capacity
5. Long-term management: Develop strategies for long-term disease control with minimal side effects

5.1.2 Treatment Considerations

1. Disease severity and extent
2. Patient preferences and expectations
3. Potential side effects and long-term safety
4. Cost and availability of treatments
5. Impact on quality of life
6. Presence of comorbidities or contraindications to specific therapies

5.2 Topical Treatments

Topical therapies are often the first-line approach for managing JLI, particularly in mild to moderate cases.

5.2.1 Topical Corticosteroids

1. Mechanisms: Anti-inflammatory and immunomodulatory effects
2. Efficacy: Moderate effectiveness, particularly for symptomatic relief
3. Usage: Usually medium to high potency steroids, applied once or twice daily
4. Considerations:

- Risk of skin atrophy with long-term use
  - Potential for tachyphylaxis

- May be more effective when used under occlusion

5.2.2 Topical Calcineurin Inhibitors

1. Agents: Tacrolimus ointment, Pimecrolimus cream
2. Mechanisms: Inhibition of T cell activation and cytokine production
3. Efficacy: Moderate effectiveness, may be particularly useful for facial lesions
4. Considerations:

- Generally well-tolerated, no risk of skin atrophy
    - May cause transient burning sensation upon application
    - Long-term safety profile is favorable

5.2.3 Topical Retinoids

1. Agents: Tretinoin, Adapalene
2. Mechanisms: Modulation of keratinocyte differentiation and immunomodulatory effects
3. Efficacy: Limited data specific to JLI, but may be helpful in some cases
4. Considerations:

- Can cause skin irritation, especially initially
    - May increase photosensitivity

5.2.4 Other Topical Agents

1. Topical vitamin D analogues (e.g., Calcipotriol): Limited data, but may have immunomodulatory effects
2. Topical antioxidants: Emerging interest, but limited evidence in JLI

5.3 Systemic Medications

In cases where topical treatments are insufficient or the disease is more extensive, systemic therapies may be considered.

5.3.1 Antimalarials

1. Agents: Hydroxychloroquine, Chloroquine
2. Mechanisms: Multiple immunomodulatory effects, including inhibition of antigen presentation
3. Efficacy: Moderate to good effectiveness in many cases, often considered first-line systemic therapy
4. Dosing: Hydroxychloroquine typically 200-400mg daily
5. Considerations:

- Slow onset of action (may take 2-3 months to see effects)
   - Requires regular ophthalmological monitoring due to rare risk of retinal toxicity
   - Generally well-tolerated, but can cause gastrointestinal side effects

5.3.2 Systemic Corticosteroids

1. Mechanisms: Potent anti-inflammatory and immunosuppressive effects
2. Efficacy: Can be highly effective for rapid control of flares
3. Usage: Usually short courses (e.g., prednisone 0.5-1 mg/kg/day for 1-2 weeks)
4. Considerations:

- Not suitable for long-term use due to side effect profile
   - Can be used as a bridge to other therapies

- Risk of rebound flare upon discontinuation

5.3.3 Methotrexate

1. Mechanism: Antiproliferative and immunomodulatory effects
2. Efficacy: Moderate effectiveness, particularly in recalcitrant cases
3. Dosing: Typically 7.5-25mg weekly
4. Considerations:

- Requires regular monitoring of blood counts and liver function
    - Contraindicated in pregnancy
    - May take several weeks to show full effect

5.3.4 Thalidomide

1. Mechanism: Immunomodulatory and anti-inflammatory effects
2. Efficacy: Reported to be effective in some refractory cases
3. Considerations:

- Significant side effect profile, including teratogenicity and peripheral neuropathy
    - Requires strict contraceptive measures
    - Generally reserved for severe, recalcitrant cases

5.3.5 Other Systemic Agents

1. Dapsone: Limited data, but may be effective in some cases
2. Cyclosporine: Used in some refractory cases, but limited long-term data
3. Mycophenolate mofetil: Emerging data suggesting potential efficacy in

resistant cases

5.4 Phototherapy Options

Light-based therapies can be effective in managing JLI, although their use must be balanced against the potential photosensitivity seen in some patients.

5.4.1 Narrowband UVB (NB-UVB)

1. Mechanism: Immunomodulatory effects on skin-resident T cells
2. Efficacy: Moderate to good effectiveness in many cases
3. Protocol: Typically 2-3 sessions per week, starting with low doses and gradually increasing
4. Considerations:

- Generally well-tolerated
   - May require maintenance therapy to prevent relapse
   - Long-term use may increase photoaging and theoretical risk of skin cancer

5.4.2 Psoralen + UVA (PUVA)

1. Mechanism: Psoralen enhances the effects of UVA on immune cells
2. Efficacy: Can be highly effective, particularly in resistant cases
3. Considerations:

- More potential side effects than NB-UVB, including nausea from psoralen and increased photosensitivity
   - Higher long-term risk of skin cancer compared to NB-UVB
   - May be used topically (bath PUVA) or systemically (oral PUVA)

5.4.3 Excimer Laser (308nm)

1. Mechanism: Targeted delivery of high-dose UVB to lesional skin
2. Efficacy: Can be effective for localized lesions
3. Considerations:

- Allows treatment of specific areas while sparing uninvolved skin
    - May require fewer sessions compared to whole-body phototherapy
    - Can be expensive and not widely available

5.5 Physical Treatments

Various physical treatment modalities have been employed in managing JLI, particularly for localized or resistant lesions.

5.5.1 Cryotherapy

1. Mechanism: Induces local tissue destruction and subsequent healing
2. Efficacy: Can be effective for small, localized lesions
3. Considerations:

- Risk of hypopigmentation, particularly in darker skin types
    - May require multiple treatments
    - Not suitable for extensive disease

5.5.2 Intralesional Corticosteroids

1. Mechanism: Delivers high concentrations of corticosteroids directly to the lesion
2. Efficacy: Can be highly effective for individual, resistant lesions

3. Considerations:

- Risk of skin atrophy and telangiectasia
    - Limited to use on a small number of lesions
    - May be particularly useful for thick or hypertrophic lesions

5.5.3 Pulsed Dye Laser

1. Mechanism: Targets blood vessels, potentially reducing inflammation
2. Efficacy: Limited data, but may be helpful in some cases, particularly for persistent erythema
3. Considerations:

- May require multiple treatments
    - Risk of purpura and rarely, scarring
    - Expensive and not widely available

5.6 Combination Therapies

Given the variable response to individual treatments, combination therapies are often employed in managing JLI.

5.6.1 Common Combinations

1. Topical treatments + Phototherapy: May enhance efficacy and allow for lower doses of phototherapy
2. Systemic antimalarials + Topical treatments: Often used as a comprehensive approach
3. Phototherapy + Systemic medications: May allow for lower doses of systemic agents

5.6.2 Sequential Therapy

In some cases, a sequential approach may be used:

1. Initial intensive therapy to induce remission (e.g., short course of systemic corticosteroids)
2. Followed by maintenance therapy with less intensive options (e.g., topical treatments or antimalarials)

5.7 Emerging and Experimental Therapies

As our understanding of JLI pathogenesis evolves, new therapeutic approaches are being explored.

5.7.1 Biologics

While not currently approved for JLI, some biologics have shown promise in case reports or small series:

1. Anti-TNF agents (e.g., etanercept, adalimumab): Limited reports of efficacy in resistant cases
2. IL-17 inhibitors (e.g., secukinumab): Theoretical potential based on the role of Th17 cells in JLI
3. JAK inhibitors (e.g., tofacitinib): Emerging interest based on their broad immunomodulatory effects

5.7.2 Other Emerging Approaches

1. Photodynamic therapy: Limited data, but may be effective in some

cases

2. Autologous platelet-rich plasma: Preliminary reports suggesting potential benefit

3. Stem cell-based therapies: Early research stage, but potential for future applications

5.8 Management of Refractory Cases

Despite the range of available treatments, some cases of JLI prove resistant to standard therapies.

5.8.1 Approach to Refractory Cases

1. Re-evaluate the diagnosis: Consider repeat biopsy or additional investigations
2. Assess adherence and optimize current therapies
3. Consider combination or rotational therapies
4. Explore less common or off-label treatments under specialist supervision
5. Consider enrollment in clinical trials of novel therapies

5.8.2 Potential Options for Refractory Cases

1. High-dose intravenous immunoglobulin (IVIG): Limited reports of efficacy in severe cases
2. Extracorporeal photopheresis: Anecdotal reports of benefit in resistant cases
3. Newer small molecule inhibitors: As they become available and are studied in related conditions

5.9 Special Considerations in JLI Management

5.9.1 Photosensitivity

For patients with photosensitive JLI:

1. Emphasize photoprotection measures
2. Consider antimalarials as they may have additional photoprotective effects
3. Cautious use of phototherapy, starting with low doses

5.9.2 Pregnancy and Lactation

1. Many systemic treatments are contraindicated in pregnancy
2. Focus on topical treatments and physical modalities where possible
3. Careful risk-benefit analysis for any systemic therapy

5.9.3 Pediatric JLI

1. Prioritize topical treatments and phototherapy where possible
2. Cautious use of systemic therapies, considering long-term safety
3. Tailor treatment approach to minimize impact on growth and development

5.9.4 Elderly Patients

1. Consider comorbidities and potential drug interactions

2. May need dose adjustments for systemic therapies
3. Increased vigilance for treatment-related side effects

5.10 Monitoring and Follow-up

Effective management of JLI requires ongoing monitoring and follow-up.

5.10.1 Assessment of Treatment Response

1. Regular clinical evaluation of lesions (size, number, symptoms)
2. Consider standardized photography for objective comparison
3. Patient-reported outcomes, including quality of life measures

5.10.2 Monitoring for Adverse Effects

1. Regular blood tests for patients on systemic therapies
2. Ophthalmological monitoring for patients on antimalarials
3. Skin examinations for patients receiving phototherapy

5.10.3 Long-term Follow-up

1. Regular follow-up intervals, adjusted based on disease activity and treatment
2. Monitoring for potential long-term complications or associated conditions
3. Adjustment of treatment plan as needed based on disease course and new evidence

5.11 Patient Education and Support

A crucial aspect of JLI management is patient education and support.

5.11.1 Key Education Points

1. Chronic nature of the condition and importance of long-term management
2. Potential triggers and exacerbating factors
3. Importance of sun protection
4. Treatment options, including benefits and potential side effects
5. Self-monitoring techniques

5.11.2 Psychological Support

1. Acknowledge the psychological impact of the condition
2. Provide resources for coping strategies
3. Consider referral for psychological support when needed

5.11.3 Lifestyle Modifications

1. Stress management techniques
2. Dietary considerations (although direct dietary links to JLI are not well-established)
3. Avoidance of potential irritants or triggers

Conclusion

The management of Jessner's Lymphocytic Infiltrate requires a personalized approach, taking into account the individual patient's disease characteristics, preferences, and response to treatment. While no single therapy is universally effective, a range of options from topical treatments to systemic medications and phototherapy allows for tailored management strategies.

As our understanding of JLI pathogenesis continues to evolve, new therapeutic targets are likely to emerge, offering hope for more effective and targeted treatments in the future. In the meantime, a comprehensive approach combining appropriate medical therapies with patient education and support remains the cornerstone of effective JLI management.

In the next chapter, we will explore management strategies for healthcare professionals, including treatment algorithms and multidisciplinary approaches to care, building upon the treatment modalities discussed here.

CHAPTER 6

anagement Strategies for Healthcare Professionals

Building upon our understanding of the various treatment modalities available for Jessner's Lymphocytic Infiltrate (JLI), this chapter focuses on comprehensive management strategies for healthcare professionals. We will explore treatment algorithms, discuss the importance of a multidisciplinary approach, and provide guidance on long-term management and follow-up protocols.

6.1 Principles of JLI Management

Before delving into specific strategies, it's crucial to establish the core principles that should guide the management of JLI:

6.1.1 Individualized Approach

Each patient with JLI presents a unique combination of disease characteristics, personal preferences, and life circumstances. Management should be tailored to:

1. Disease severity and extent
2. Impact on quality of life
3. Patient's age and overall health status

4. Personal preferences and treatment goals
5. Accessibility and affordability of treatment options

6.1.2 Shared Decision-Making

Involve patients in treatment decisions by:

1. Educating them about their condition and available treatment options
2. Discussing potential benefits and risks of each approach
3. Considering their personal goals and preferences
4. Encouraging active participation in their care plan

6.1.3 Step-wise Approach

Generally, a step-wise approach to treatment is recommended:

1. Start with less aggressive treatments (e.g., topical therapies)
2. Progress to more intensive options if needed
3. Consider combination therapies for optimal management
4. Adjust treatment based on response and tolerability

6.1.4 Long-term Perspective

Given the chronic nature of JLI, management should focus on:

1. Long-term disease control
2. Minimizing cumulative treatment-related side effects

3. Maintaining quality of life
4. Regular monitoring and follow-up

6.2 Treatment Algorithms

While treatment must be individualized, algorithms can provide a helpful framework for approaching JLI management.

6.2.1 Initial Evaluation

1. Confirm diagnosis through clinical assessment and biopsy
2. Assess disease severity and extent
3. Evaluate impact on quality of life
4. Screen for associated conditions or complications
5. Identify any contraindications to specific treatments

6.2.2 Mild to Moderate Localized Disease

First-line:

1. Topical corticosteroids (medium to high potency)
2. Topical calcineurin inhibitors (especially for facial lesions)

If inadequate response after 4-6 weeks:

1. Consider intralesional corticosteroids for resistant lesions
2. Trial of phototherapy (NB-UVB or excimer laser)

If still inadequate:

1. Consider systemic therapy (e.g., antimalarials)
2. Referral to dermatology if not already involved

6.2.3 Moderate to Severe or Widespread Disease

First-line:

1. Systemic antimalarials (e.g., hydroxychloroquine)
2. Concurrent use of topical treatments

If inadequate response after 2-3 months:

1. Add phototherapy (NB-UVB)
2. Consider short course of systemic corticosteroids for acute flares

If still inadequate:

1. Consider alternative systemic therapies (e.g., methotrexate, dapsone)
2. Evaluate for combination therapies

6.2.4 Refractory Disease

For cases resistant to standard therapies:

1. Re-evaluate diagnosis and consider repeat biopsy
2. Consider more aggressive systemic therapies (e.g., thalidomide, under specialist supervision)

3. Explore experimental or off-label treatments
4. Evaluate for clinical trial eligibility

6.2.5 Maintenance Therapy

Once disease control is achieved:

1. Gradually taper treatments to lowest effective dose
2. Consider intermittent or rotational therapy to minimize side effects
3. Maintain vigilant photoprotection

6.3 Multidisciplinary Approach to Care

Effective management of JLI often requires a multidisciplinary approach, particularly in complex or refractory cases.

6.3.1 Core Team Members

1. Dermatologist: Central to diagnosis and management
2. Primary Care Physician: Coordinates overall care and manages comorbidities
3. Dermatopathologist: Crucial for accurate diagnosis and monitoring

6.3.2 Additional Specialists

Depending on individual patient needs:

1. Rheumatologist: For cases with features overlapping with connective tissue diseases

2. Ophthalmologist: For monitoring patients on antimalarials
3. Psychiatrist or Psychologist: To address psychological impact
4. Pain Specialist: In cases with significant symptomatic burden
5. Clinical Immunologist: For complex cases or when considering novel immunomodulatory therapies

6.3.3 Allied Health Professionals

1. Nurse Specialists: Patient education and treatment administration
2. Pharmacists: Medication counseling and monitoring
3. Occupational Therapists: For cases impacting daily activities
4. Dietitians: Advice on anti-inflammatory diets, though direct dietary links to JLI are not well-established

6.3.4 Coordinating Care

Effective multidisciplinary care requires:

1. Clear communication channels between team members
2. Regular case discussions or multidisciplinary team meetings for complex cases
3. Shared electronic health records where possible
4. Designated care coordinator (often the dermatologist or primary care physician)

6.4 Monitoring and Follow-up Protocols

Systematic monitoring and follow-up are crucial for effective long-term management of JLI.

6.4.1 Initial Follow-up

After starting a new treatment:

1. First follow-up at 4-6 weeks to assess initial response and tolerability
2. Adjust treatment as needed based on response and side effects

6.4.2 Routine Follow-up

For stable patients:

1. Every 3-6 months initially
2. Can be extended to every 6-12 months for well-controlled disease
3. More frequent visits for active disease or when adjusting treatments

6.4.3 Monitoring Disease Activity

At each visit:

1. Assess extent and severity of lesions
2. Evaluate symptomatic burden (e.g., pruritus, burning sensation)
3. Review patient-reported outcomes and quality of life measures
4. Consider standardized photography for objective comparison

6.4.4 Treatment-Specific Monitoring

Tailor monitoring based on specific treatments:

1. Topical steroids: Monitor for skin atrophy, telangiectasia
2. Antimalarials: Regular ophthalmological exams (baseline, then annually

after 5 years, or sooner in high-risk patients)
3. Methotrexate: Regular blood counts, liver function tests
4. Phototherapy: Regular skin examinations, cumulative dose tracking

6.4.5 Long-term Complications

Monitor for potential long-term issues:

1. Cumulative effects of treatments (e.g., skin aging with phototherapy)
2. Development of associated autoimmune conditions
3. Psychological impact of chronic disease

6.5 Patient Education and Self-Management

Empowering patients through education and self-management strategies is key to successful long-term management.

6.5.1 Disease Education

Provide comprehensive information on:

1. Nature of JLI and its expected course
2. Treatment options and their rationale
3. Importance of adherence to treatment plans
4. Potential triggers and exacerbating factors

6.5.2 Self-Monitoring Techniques

Teach patients to:

1. Recognize signs of disease flare
2. Identify potential treatment-related side effects
3. Keep a symptom diary if helpful

6.5.3 Lifestyle Management

Guide patients on:

1. Sun protection strategies
2. Stress management techniques
3. Appropriate skincare routines

6.5.4 When to Seek Medical Attention

Instruct patients to seek care for:

1. Sudden worsening of symptoms
2. Development of new or unusual symptoms
3. Suspected treatment-related side effects

6.6 Managing Comorbidities and Special Situations

JLI management may be complicated by comorbidities or special circumstances that require careful consideration.

6.6.1 Cardiovascular Risk

While JLI itself is not associated with increased cardiovascular risk:

1. Some treatments (e.g., systemic corticosteroids) may impact cardiovas-

cular health

2. Regular cardiovascular risk assessment and management is advisable

6.6.2 Pregnancy and Family Planning

For patients considering pregnancy:

1. Discuss treatment options well in advance
2. Adjust medications as needed (many systemic treatments are contraindicated)
3. Develop a management plan for during and after pregnancy

6.6.3 Pediatric and Adolescent Patients

In younger patients:

1. Consider impact of treatments on growth and development
2. Address psychosocial aspects, particularly body image concerns
3. Involve parents/guardians in treatment decisions and management

6.6.4 Elderly Patients

In older patients:

1. Consider comorbidities and potential drug interactions
2. Adjust treatment doses as needed, particularly for systemic therapies
3. Be vigilant for treatment-related side effects

6.7 Managing Treatment Failures and Refractory Disease

Despite optimal management, some cases of JLI prove difficult to control, requiring a systematic approach.

6.7.1 Assessing Treatment Failure

Before labeling a case as refractory:

1. Ensure correct diagnosis (consider repeat biopsy if needed)
2. Assess treatment adherence
3. Evaluate for exacerbating factors (e.g., undisclosed sun exposure)
4. Consider if sufficient time has been allowed for treatment response

6.7.2 Strategies for Refractory Disease

1. Combination therapies: Combine treatments with different mechanisms of action
2. Rotational therapy: Cycle through different treatments to prevent tachyphylaxis
3. Dose escalation: Increase doses of current treatments if tolerated
4. Novel or off-label therapies: Consider under specialist supervision
5. Clinical trials: Evaluate eligibility for ongoing studies of new treatments

6.7.3 Referral to Specialized Centers

Consider referral to specialized centers for:

1. Access to advanced or experimental therapies
2. Multidisciplinary care for complex cases
3. Participation in clinical trials

6.8 Incorporating New Evidence into Practice

The field of dermatology is rapidly evolving, and management strategies for JLI should be updated as new evidence emerges.

6.8.1 Staying Informed

Healthcare professionals should:

1. Regularly review current literature on JLI
2. Attend relevant conferences and continuing education events
3. Participate in professional networks or forums focused on cutaneous immunology

6.8.2 Evaluating New Treatments

When considering new treatments:

1. Critically appraise the available evidence
2. Consider the risk-benefit profile in the context of existing therapies
3. Start with a limited trial in appropriate patients
4. Monitor and document outcomes carefully

6.8.3 Updating Treatment Protocols

Periodically review and update treatment protocols based on:

1. New clinical evidence
2. Updated guidelines from professional societies
3. Local experience and patient outcomes

6.9 Quality Improvement in JLI Management

Implementing quality improvement initiatives can enhance the overall management of JLI patients.

6.9.1 Audit and Feedback

Regularly audit clinical practices:

1. Treatment outcomes
2. Adherence to follow-up protocols
3. Patient satisfaction

Use audit results to inform practice improvements.

6.9.2 Standardized Care Pathways

Develop and implement standardized care pathways:

1. Ensure consistent high-quality care
2. Facilitate smooth transitions between healthcare providers
3. Incorporate decision support tools where appropriate

6.9.3 Patient-Reported Outcome Measures

Incorporate validated patient-reported outcome measures:

1. Assess impact on quality of life
2. Evaluate treatment satisfaction
3. Use results to guide management decisions

6.9.4 Continuous Professional Development

Encourage ongoing education and training:

1. Regular case discussions or journal clubs
2. Skill development workshops (e.g., for performing biopsies or administering treatments)
3. Cross-training to ensure comprehensive care

6.10 Ethical Considerations in JLI Management

Healthcare professionals should be aware of ethical considerations in managing JLI:

6.10.1 Informed Consent

Ensure patients are fully informed about:

1. Nature of their condition
2. Available treatment options
3. Potential risks and benefits of each treatment
4. Any off-label use of medications

6.10.2 Resource Allocation

Balance individual patient needs with broader resource considerations:

1. Cost-effective use of treatments
2. Equitable access to care
3. Appropriate use of specialist services

6.10.3 Research Ethics

When involving patients in research:

1. Ensure proper informed consent
2. Maintain patient privacy and confidentiality
3. Balance research goals with patient care priorities

Conclusion

Effective management of Jessner's Lymphocytic Infiltrate requires a comprehensive, patient-centered approach that goes beyond simply prescribing treatments. By implementing structured treatment algorithms, fostering multidisciplinary collaboration, maintaining rigorous monitoring protocols, and empowering patients through education and self-management strategies, healthcare professionals can optimize outcomes for individuals living with JLI.

The chronic and sometimes unpredictable nature of JLI necessitates a long-term perspective in management, with an emphasis on maintaining disease control while minimizing cumulative treatment-related side effects. Flexibility in approach, willingness to adjust strategies based on patient response, and openness to incorporating new evidence as it emerges are key to successful management.

As our understanding of JLI continues to evolve, so too will our management strategies. By staying informed of the latest developments, critically evaluating new evidence, and continuously striving to improve the quality of care provided, healthcare professionals can ensure that patients with JLI receive the best possible management, enhancing their quality of life and long-term outcomes.

In the next chapter, we will explore the patient perspective on living with Jessner's Lymphocytic Infiltrate, providing valuable insights that can further inform and enhance our management approaches.

CHAPTER 7

L iving with Jessner's Lymphocytic Infiltrate: Patient Perspectives

Understanding the patient experience is crucial for providing comprehensive care for individuals with Jessner's Lymphocytic Infiltrate (JLI). This chapter explores the daily realities, challenges, and coping strategies of those living with JLI, offering valuable insights for both healthcare professionals and patients.

7.1 The Journey to Diagnosis

The path to a JLI diagnosis can be complex and often frustrating for patients.

7.1.1 Initial Symptoms and Concerns

Patients often report:

1. Confusion and worry about unexplained skin lesions
2. Frustration with the appearance of persistent rashes
3. Concerns about potential serious underlying conditions

7.1.2 Seeking Medical Attention

Common experiences include:

1. Multiple visits to different healthcare providers
2. Misdiagnoses or tentative diagnoses before reaching a definitive JLI diagnosis
3. Feelings of relief mixed with anxiety upon finally receiving a diagnosis

7.1.3 Patient Narrative: The Diagnostic Journey

"When I first noticed the red patches on my face, I thought it was just a temporary rash. But as weeks turned into months, and the lesions didn't go away, I began to worry. I saw my primary care doctor, who referred me to a dermatologist. Even then, it took several visits and a biopsy before I was diagnosed with JLI. The process was frustrating, but I felt relieved to finally have a name for what was happening to my skin." - Sarah, JLI patient for 5 years

7.2 Physical Impact of JLI

While JLI is not life-threatening, it can have significant physical effects on patients.

7.2.1 Skin Manifestations

Patients describe:

1. Visible redness and raised lesions, particularly distressing on the face
2. Variations in appearance over time, with periods of improvement and flare-ups
3. Concerns about permanent skin changes or scarring

7.2.2 Associated Symptoms

Common physical experiences include:

1. Itching or burning sensations in affected areas
2. Sensitivity to touch in lesional skin
3. Photosensitivity in some cases, limiting sun exposure

7.2.3 Impact on Daily Activities

JLI can affect:

1. Sleep, if lesions are symptomatic
2. Choice of clothing, to cover affected areas
3. Participation in outdoor activities, especially for photosensitive individuals

7.3 Psychological and Emotional Impact

The visible nature of JLI can have profound psychological effects on patients.

7.3.1 Body Image and Self-esteem

Many patients report:

1. Decreased self-confidence, especially when lesions are on visible areas
2. Feelings of self-consciousness in social situations
3. Concerns about attractiveness and how others perceive them

7.3.2 Emotional Responses

Common emotional experiences include:

1. Frustration with the chronic and unpredictable nature of JLI
2. Anxiety about potential flare-ups or worsening of the condition
3. Sadness or depression related to the impact on quality of life

7.3.3 Patient Narrative: Emotional Journey

"There are days when I look in the mirror and barely recognize myself. The red patches on my face make me feel like hiding away. I've had to work hard on accepting this condition and not letting it define me. It's been an emotional rollercoaster, but I'm learning to focus on the things I can control and finding ways to boost my self-esteem despite JLI." - Mark, living with JLI for 8 years

7.4 Social and Relationship Impacts

JLI can significantly affect patients' social lives and relationships.

7.4.1 Social Interactions

Patients often experience:

1. Reluctance to engage in social activities during flare-ups
2. Difficulty explaining their condition to others
3. Unwanted attention or questions about their appearance

7.4.2 Intimate Relationships

JLI can impact:

1. Dating and forming new romantic relationships
2. Intimacy in established relationships

3. Concerns about genetic factors if considering starting a family

7.4.3 Family Dynamics

Families of JLI patients may experience:

1. Worry and concern for their loved one
2. Need for education about the condition
3. Adjustments to family activities or routines to accommodate the patient's needs

7.5 Professional and Financial Impacts

Living with JLI can have implications for patients' professional lives and finances.

7.5.1 Workplace Challenges

Patients may face:

1. Difficulty in customer-facing roles, especially during flare-ups
2. Need for workplace accommodations (e.g., avoiding certain lighting or allowing flexible hours for medical appointments)
3. Concerns about job security or career advancement

7.5.2 Financial Burden

JLI can lead to:

1. High costs of treatments, especially for uninsured or underinsured

patients

2. Lost work time due to medical appointments or severe flare-ups
3. Expenses for cosmetics or clothing to conceal lesions

7.5.3 Patient Narrative: Professional Impact

"As a sales representative, my appearance is a big part of my job. When my JLI flares up, it affects my confidence in client meetings. I've had to be upfront with my employer about my condition. Fortunately, they've been understanding, allowing me to do more behind-the-scenes work during bad flare-ups. Still, I worry about the long-term impact on my career." - David, diagnosed with JLI 3 years ago

7.6 Coping Strategies and Lifestyle Adjustments

Patients with JLI develop various strategies to manage their condition and its impacts.

7.6.1 Skincare and Cosmetic Approaches

Many patients adopt:

1. Specialized skincare routines to manage symptoms and appearance
2. Use of cosmetics to conceal lesions
3. Clothing choices to cover affected areas when desired

7.6.2 Stress Management

Common strategies include:

1. Mindfulness and meditation practices

2. Regular exercise, adapted as needed for skin comfort
3. Engaging in hobbies or activities that promote relaxation

7.6.3 Dietary Approaches

While direct dietary links to JLI are not well-established, some patients report benefits from:

1. Anti-inflammatory diets
2. Avoiding potential trigger foods (individually identified)
3. Maintaining overall good nutrition

7.6.4 Patient Narrative: Lifestyle Adaptations

"Living with JLI has prompted me to make some positive changes in my life. I've become more conscious about sun protection, not just for my JLI but for overall skin health. I've also found that regular yoga and meditation help me manage stress, which seems to reduce my flare-ups. It's been a journey of self-discovery in many ways." - Lisa, JLI patient for 6 years

7.7 Treatment Experiences and Challenges

Patients' experiences with JLI treatments can vary widely.

7.7.1 Treatment Efficacy

Patients often report:

1. Variability in response to different treatments
2. Frustration with trial-and-error approaches to find effective therapies
3. Periods of improvement followed by unexpected flare-ups

7.7.2 Side Effects and Tolerability

Common experiences include:

1. Concerns about long-term use of medications, especially systemic treatments
2. Balancing treatment efficacy with side effect profiles
3. Challenges in adhering to complex treatment regimens

7.7.3 Access to Care

Patients may face:

1. Difficulty finding healthcare providers experienced with JLI
2. Long wait times for specialist appointments
3. Geographical barriers to accessing specialized treatments

7.7.4 Patient Narrative: Treatment Journey

"I've tried so many treatments over the years - creams, pills, light therapy. Some worked for a while, then seemed to lose effectiveness. The side effects were challenging at times, especially with the stronger medications. It's been a process of constantly adjusting and trying to find the right balance. I'm grateful for my dermatologist who has been patient and persistent in finding the best approach for me." - Robert, living with JLI for 10 years

7.8 Support Systems and Resources

Support plays a crucial role in helping patients cope with JLI.

7.8.1 Family and Friends

Patients often rely on:

1. Emotional support from close family and friends
2. Practical help during severe flare-ups
3. Understanding and accommodation of their needs

7.8.2 Patient Support Groups

Many find value in:

1. Connecting with others who have JLI
2. Sharing experiences and coping strategies
3. Feeling less isolated in their experience

7.8.3 Online Resources

Patients frequently use:

1. Online forums and social media groups for JLI
2. Reputable websites for medical information
3. Blogs or vlogs by other JLI patients

7.8.4 Patient Narrative: Finding Support

"Joining an online support group for JLI was a turning point for me. Suddenly, I wasn't alone in this. Hearing others' stories, sharing tips, and just knowing there are people who truly understand what I'm going through has been incredibly comforting. It's become a valuable part of my support system." - Emily, diagnosed with JLI 4 years ago

7.9 Hopes and Concerns for the Future

Patients with JLI often have mixed feelings about their future with the condition.

7.9.1 Hopes

Common aspirations include:

1. Development of more effective treatments
2. Better understanding of JLI's causes, potentially leading to prevention
3. Increased public awareness and understanding of the condition

7.9.2 Concerns

Frequent worries involve:

1. Long-term health impacts of JLI or its treatments
2. Potential for the condition to worsen over time
3. Impact on future life plans (career, relationships, etc.)

7.9.3 Patient Narrative: Looking Ahead

"Sometimes I worry about what JLI means for my future. Will it get worse as I get older? Will there be better treatments? But I also have hope. I've learned so much about taking care of myself, and I'm optimistic that research will lead to new breakthroughs. In the meantime, I'm focusing on living my best life, JLI and all." - Michael, JLI patient for 7 years

7.10 Advice from Patients to Healthcare Providers

Patients often have valuable insights for improving care.

7.10.1 Communication

Patients appreciate:

1. Clear, jargon-free explanations of their condition and treatments
2. Active listening and validation of their experiences
3. Openness to discussing alternative or complementary approaches

7.10.2 Personalized Care

Patients value:

1. Recognition of the individual nature of JLI and its impacts
2. Willingness to adjust treatment plans based on patient feedback
3. Consideration of quality of life in treatment decisions

7.10.3 Holistic Approach

Many patients seek:

1. Attention to both physical and psychological aspects of JLI
2. Guidance on lifestyle factors (diet, stress management, etc.)
3. Help in accessing additional resources or support services

7.10.4 Patient Narrative: Message to Providers

"To healthcare providers treating JLI patients, please remember that this condition affects more than just our skin. It impacts every aspect of our lives. We need your medical expertise, but we also need your empathy and understanding. Partner with us in our care, listen to our concerns, and help us find ways to live well despite JLI." - Karen, living with JLI for 9 years

7.11 The Role of Patient Advocacy

Patient advocacy plays an important role in improving care and awareness for JLI.

7.11.1 Raising Awareness

Patient advocates work towards:

1. Increasing public understanding of JLI
2. Reducing stigma associated with visible skin conditions
3. Promoting research into JLI causes and treatments

7.11.2 Improving Care

Advocacy efforts focus on:

1. Ensuring access to appropriate treatments
2. Promoting patient-centered care approaches
3. Encouraging the development of clinical guidelines for JLI management

7.11.3 Supporting Research

Patients contribute to research through:

1. Participation in clinical trials
2. Sharing their experiences for qualitative studies

3. Fundraising for JLI research initiatives

Conclusion

Living with Jessner's Lymphocytic Infiltrate presents numerous challenges that extend far beyond the physical manifestations of the condition. Patients navigate a complex journey from diagnosis through treatment, all while managing the significant impacts on their psychological well-being, social interactions, and professional lives.

The experiences shared in this chapter highlight the resilience and adaptability of individuals living with JLI. From developing personalized coping strategies to advocating for better care and understanding, these patients offer valuable insights that can inform and improve the management of JLI.

For healthcare providers, understanding the patient perspective is crucial for delivering compassionate, effective, and holistic care. By recognizing the full spectrum of JLI's impacts and working collaboratively with patients, providers can help individuals not just manage their condition, but thrive despite its challenges.

As research continues and our understanding of JLI evolves, the hope is that these patient experiences will drive improvements in diagnosis, treatment, and support, ultimately enhancing the quality of life for all those affected by Jessner's Lymphocytic Infiltrate.

The next chapter will explore the psychological impact of JLI in greater depth, examining the mental health considerations and support strategies crucial for comprehensive patient care.

CHAPTER 8

Psychological Impact and Support

The psychological impact of Jessner's Lymphocytic Infiltrate (JLI) is a crucial aspect of the condition that requires careful consideration and management. This chapter delves into the mental health implications of living with JLI, explores various psychological support strategies, and discusses the importance of a holistic approach to patient care.

8.1 Understanding the Psychological Burden of JLI

Living with a chronic, visible skin condition like JLI can have profound psychological effects on patients.

8.1.1 Common Psychological Challenges

Patients with JLI often experience:

1. Anxiety related to the unpredictable nature of flare-ups
2. Depression stemming from the chronic nature of the condition
3. Social anxiety, particularly in situations where their skin is visible
4. Body image issues and lowered self-esteem
5. Frustration and anger about the impact of JLI on their lives

8.1.2 Factors Influencing Psychological Impact

The severity of psychological distress can vary based on:

1. Visibility and extent of skin lesions
2. Individual personality traits and coping mechanisms
3. Level of social support
4. Impact on daily activities and quality of life
5. Effectiveness of treatments and management strategies

8.1.3 The Cycle of Stress and Skin Symptoms

Many patients report a bidirectional relationship between stress and JLI symptoms:

1. Stress can exacerbate skin symptoms
2. Worsening skin symptoms can increase psychological distress
3. This cycle can lead to a negative feedback loop, impacting both mental health and skin condition

8.2 Assessing Psychological Well-being in JLI Patients

Regular assessment of psychological well-being is crucial for comprehensive care of JLI patients.

8.2.1 Screening Tools

Healthcare providers can utilize various screening tools:

1. Dermatology Life Quality Index (DLQI) for assessing quality of life impact

2. Hospital Anxiety and Depression Scale (HADS) for detecting anxiety and depression
3. Body Image Quality of Life Inventory (BIQLI) for evaluating body image concerns

8.2.2 Clinical Interview Techniques

Effective assessment often involves:

1. Open-ended questions about the emotional impact of JLI
2. Inquiries about changes in mood, sleep patterns, and social interactions
3. Exploration of the patient's coping strategies and support systems

8.2.3 Red Flags for Serious Mental Health Concerns

Healthcare providers should be alert to signs of:

1. Clinical depression, including persistent low mood and loss of interest in activities
2. Severe anxiety interfering with daily functioning
3. Social isolation or withdrawal
4. Body dysmorphic tendencies related to skin appearance
5. Suicidal ideation or self-harm behaviors

8.3 Common Psychological Disorders Associated with JLI

While not all patients with JLI will develop mental health disorders, some are at increased risk for certain conditions.

8.3.1 Depression

Characteristics in JLI patients may include:

1. Persistent sadness or hopelessness about their condition
2. Loss of interest in previously enjoyed activities
3. Sleep disturbances, often exacerbated by skin symptoms
4. Feelings of worthlessness related to appearance

8.3.2 Anxiety Disorders

Common manifestations include:

1. Generalized anxiety about the course of JLI and its treatment
2. Social anxiety, particularly in situations where skin is exposed
3. Panic attacks triggered by sudden flare-ups or social situations

8.3.3 Body Dysmorphic Disorder (BDD)

While distinct from JLI, some patients may develop BDD-like symptoms:

1. Excessive preoccupation with perceived flaws in appearance
2. Repetitive behaviors (e.g., mirror checking, excessive grooming)
3. Significant distress and functional impairment due to appearance concerns

8.3.4 Adjustment Disorders

Some patients may experience:

1. Difficulty adapting to the diagnosis of a chronic condition
2. Challenges in coping with lifestyle changes necessitated by JLI

8.4 Psychological Support Strategies

A range of psychological support strategies can be beneficial for patients with JLI.

8.4.1 Cognitive Behavioral Therapy (CBT)

CBT can help patients:

1. Identify and challenge negative thought patterns about their appearance
2. Develop coping strategies for managing stress and anxiety
3. Improve problem-solving skills for dealing with JLI-related challenges

8.4.2 Mindfulness and Relaxation Techniques

These approaches can assist in:

1. Reducing stress and its potential impact on skin symptoms
2. Improving overall emotional well-being
3. Enhancing body awareness and acceptance

8.4.3 Support Groups

Participation in support groups offers:

1. Opportunities to connect with others facing similar challenges
2. Sharing of coping strategies and practical tips
3. Reduction of feelings of isolation and stigma

8.4.4 Art Therapy and Expressive Arts

Creative approaches can provide:

1. Non-verbal outlets for expressing emotions related to JLI
2. Opportunities for self-discovery and personal growth
3. Improved self-esteem through creative accomplishment

8.5 The Role of Psychodermatology

Psychodermatology, an emerging field at the intersection of dermatology and psychology, offers a specialized approach to caring for patients with skin conditions like JLI.

8.5.1 Principles of Psychodermatology

Key concepts include:

1. Recognition of the bi-directional relationship between skin and mind
2. Integration of psychological interventions into dermatological care
3. Holistic approach addressing both physical and emotional aspects of skin conditions

8.5.2 Psychodermatological Interventions

Specialized interventions may include:

1. Combined consultations with dermatologists and mental health professionals
2. Tailored psychological therapies addressing skin-related distress
3. Mind-body interventions specifically designed for dermatology patients

8.5.3 Benefits of a Psychodermatological Approach

This integrated approach can lead to:

1. Improved treatment adherence and outcomes
2. Enhanced patient satisfaction with care
3. More comprehensive management of both skin symptoms and related psychological distress

8.6 Enhancing Resilience and Coping Skills

Building resilience and effective coping skills is crucial for long-term psychological well-being in JLI patients.

8.6.1 Developing a Positive Self-Image

Strategies may include:

1. Focusing on personal strengths and achievements unrelated to appearance
2. Practicing self-compassion and challenging self-critical thoughts
3. Engaging in activities that boost self-esteem and confidence

8.6.2 Stress Management Techniques

Effective approaches often involve:

1. Regular practice of relaxation techniques (e.g., deep breathing, progressive muscle relaxation)
2. Time management and prioritization to reduce daily stressors
3. Engaging in regular physical activity, adapted as needed for skin

comfort

8.6.3 Building a Support Network

Patients can benefit from:

1. Cultivating supportive relationships with family and friends
2. Connecting with other JLI patients through support groups or online communities
3. Developing a collaborative relationship with their healthcare team

8.7 Addressing Body Image Concerns

Body image issues are common among JLI patients and require specific attention.

8.7.1 Cognitive Restructuring

Techniques may include:

1. Challenging unrealistic beauty standards and negative self-talk
2. Developing a more balanced and compassionate view of one's appearance
3. Focusing on body functionality rather than just appearance

8.7.2 Exposure Therapy

Gradual exposure can help in:

1. Reducing anxiety in situations where skin is visible

2. Building confidence in social interactions
3. Challenging avoidance behaviors that reinforce anxiety

8.7.3 Cosmetic Camouflage Techniques

While not a psychological intervention per se, learning effective camouflage techniques can:

1. Provide a sense of control over appearance
2. Reduce anxiety in social situations
3. Serve as a stepping stone towards greater acceptance

8.8 Supporting Patients Through Different Life Stages

The psychological impact of JLI can vary across different life stages, requiring tailored support.

8.8.1 Adolescents and Young Adults

Specific concerns may include:

1. Impact on emerging self-identity and self-esteem
2. Challenges in dating and forming romantic relationships
3. Career concerns, especially in appearance-focused industries

8.8.2 Adults in Mid-life

Issues might involve:

1. Balancing JLI management with family and career responsibilities

2. Concerns about aging and the long-term course of JLI
3. Impact on intimate relationships and family dynamics

8.8.3 Older Adults

Considerations may include:

1. Adjusting to changes in appearance due to both JLI and aging
2. Managing JLI alongside other health conditions
3. Maintaining independence and quality of life

8.9 The Role of Family and Partners

The support of family members and partners is crucial for the psychological well-being of JLI patients.

8.9.1 Education for Family Members

Providing families with information about:

1. The nature of JLI and its psychological impacts
2. Ways to provide effective emotional support
3. The importance of maintaining normalcy and avoiding over-focus on the condition

8.9.2 Couples Counseling

May be beneficial for:

1. Addressing intimacy concerns related to JLI

2. Improving communication about the impact of JLI on the relationship
3. Developing shared coping strategies

8.9.3 Family Therapy

Can be helpful in:

1. Addressing family dynamics affected by JLI
2. Developing a supportive family environment
3. Helping children cope with a parent's or sibling's JLI

8.10 Workplace and Career Support

JLI can have significant impacts on patients' professional lives, requiring specific psychological support.

8.10.1 Career Counseling

May involve:

1. Exploring career options compatible with managing JLI
2. Developing strategies for workplace success despite JLI challenges
3. Building confidence in professional abilities beyond appearance

8.10.2 Workplace Accommodations

Psychologists can assist in:

1. Helping patients advocate for needed accommodations
2. Developing strategies for managing JLI in the workplace

3. Addressing concerns about disclosure of the condition to employers or colleagues

8.10.3 Managing Workplace Stress

Strategies might include:

1. Techniques for managing stress in high-pressure work environments
2. Balancing work responsibilities with JLI management
3. Building resilience in the face of workplace challenges

8.11 Leveraging Technology for Psychological Support

Emerging technologies offer new avenues for providing psychological support to JLI patients.

8.11.1 Telepsychology

Benefits include:

1. Increased access to mental health support, especially for patients in remote areas
2. Convenience for patients with mobility issues or busy schedules
3. Option for more frequent, shorter check-ins

8.11.2 Mobile Apps and Digital Tools

Can provide:

1. Mood tracking and symptom monitoring

2. Guided relaxation and mindfulness exercises
3. Cognitive behavioral therapy modules tailored for skin condition-related distress

8.11.3 Virtual Reality (VR) Therapy

Emerging applications include:

1. Exposure therapy for social anxiety related to skin appearance
2. Relaxation and stress reduction in immersive environments
3. Body image interventions using VR technology

8.12 Addressing Stigma and Social Misconceptions

Psychological interventions can help patients deal with societal stigma and misconceptions about JLI.

8.12.1 Stigma Resistance Training

Techniques may include:

1. Educating patients about the nature of stigma and its impacts
2. Developing skills for addressing misconceptions about JLI
3. Building resilience against internalized stigma

8.12.2 Social Skills Training

Can help in:

1. Improving confidence in social interactions

2. Developing strategies for addressing questions or comments about JLI
3. Enhancing overall social competence and assertiveness

8.12.3 Advocacy and Empowerment

Encouraging patients to:

1. Participate in awareness-raising activities about JLI
2. Share their experiences to educate others
3. Engage in peer support and mentoring of newly diagnosed patients

8.13 Integrating Psychological Care into Overall JLI Management

For optimal patient outcomes, psychological care should be seamlessly integrated into the overall management of JLI.

8.13.1 Collaborative Care Models

Implementing models that involve:

1. Regular communication between dermatologists and mental health professionals
2. Integrated treatment plans addressing both physical and psychological aspects of JLI
3. Shared decision-making involving the patient, dermatologist, and mental health provider

8.13.2 Routine Psychological Screening

Incorporating:

1. Regular assessments of psychological well-being as part of routine JLI follow-ups
2. Use of standardized screening tools to track psychological status over time
3. Clear pathways for referral to mental health services when needed

8.13.3 Patient Education

Ensuring that patients are informed about:

1. The potential psychological impacts of JLI
2. Available support resources and interventions
3. The importance of addressing both physical and emotional aspects of living with JLI

Conclusion

The psychological impact of Jessner's Lymphocytic Infiltrate is significant and multifaceted, affecting various aspects of patients' lives from self-image and relationships to career and overall quality of life. Recognizing and addressing these psychological dimensions is crucial for providing comprehensive care to individuals with JLI.

A range of psychological support strategies, from cognitive behavioral therapy and mindfulness techniques to support groups and emerging technological interventions, can be invaluable in helping patients cope with the challenges of living with JLI. The field of psychodermatology offers a particularly promising approach, integrating dermatological and psychological care for a truly holistic treatment model.

Healthcare providers caring for JLI patients should be attuned to the psychological aspects of the condition, regularly assessing mental health status and providing or referring for appropriate support. By addressing both the physical and psychological dimensions of JLI, we can help patients not just manage their condition, but thrive despite its challenges.

As research in this area continues to evolve, we can anticipate more refined and effective approaches to supporting the psychological well-being of individuals with JLI. This integrated approach to care, addressing both skin and mind, holds the promise of significantly improving outcomes and quality of life for those living with Jessner's Lymphocytic Infiltrate.

CHAPTER 9

Jessner's Lymphocytic Infiltrate in Special Populations

While Jessner's Lymphocytic Infiltrate (JLI) primarily affects adults, it can occur in various special populations, each presenting unique challenges in diagnosis, management, and patient care. This chapter explores JLI in pediatric cases, during pregnancy and lactation, and in elderly patients, highlighting the specific considerations and approaches needed for these groups.

9.1 Pediatric Jessner's Lymphocytic Infiltrate

Although less common, JLI can occur in children and adolescents, presenting distinct challenges in diagnosis and management.

9.1.1 Epidemiology and Clinical Presentation

Pediatric JLI is rare, with key features including:

1. Typical onset in late childhood or adolescence
2. Similar clinical presentation to adult JLI, with erythematous papules and plaques
3. Potential for more widespread distribution compared to adult cases
4. Possible association with other autoimmune or inflammatory conditions in some cases

9.1.2 Diagnostic Challenges

Diagnosing JLI in pediatric patients can be challenging due to:

1. Rarity of the condition in this age group, leading to potential misdiagnosis
2. Overlap with other childhood dermatoses
3. Difficulty in obtaining biopsies in younger children
4. Need for careful differentiation from other lymphocytic infiltrates, including cutaneous lymphoma

9.1.3 Treatment Considerations

Managing pediatric JLI requires special attention to:

1. Safety and long-term effects of treatments in growing children
2. Impact on growth and development
3. Psychosocial effects of a chronic skin condition during formative years
4. Compliance issues unique to pediatric patients

9.1.4 Specific Treatment Approaches

Treatment strategies may include:

1. Topical corticosteroids as first-line therapy, with careful monitoring for side effects
2. Topical calcineurin inhibitors, particularly for facial lesions
3. Cautious use of systemic therapies, reserving them for severe or recalcitrant cases
4. Phototherapy, considering cumulative UV exposure over the patient's lifetime

5. Emphasis on non-pharmacological approaches, including rigorous sun protection

9.1.5 Long-term Prognosis and Follow-up

Considerations for long-term management include:

1. Regular follow-up to monitor disease progression and treatment response
2. Transition planning as the patient moves from pediatric to adult care
3. Monitoring for potential associated conditions that may develop over time
4. Psychosocial support throughout childhood and adolescence

9.1.6 Case Study: Pediatric JLI

"Sarah, a 14-year-old girl, presented with a 6-month history of persistent, asymptomatic erythematous plaques on her cheeks and forehead. Initial misdiagnosis as acne led to ineffective treatments. Skin biopsy confirmed JLI. Treatment with topical tacrolimus and careful sun protection led to significant improvement. Ongoing management focuses on minimizing flares and addressing the psychosocial impact of the condition during her teenage years."

9.2 Jessner's Lymphocytic Infiltrate in Pregnancy and Lactation

The management of JLI during pregnancy and lactation presents unique challenges, requiring careful consideration of maternal and fetal well-being.

9.2.1 Effects of Pregnancy on JLI

Pregnancy can impact JLI in various ways:

1. Some patients experience improvement during pregnancy due to natural immunomodulation
2. Others may see worsening or new onset of JLI, possibly related to hormonal changes
3. Postpartum period may be associated with flares in some cases

9.2.2 Diagnostic Considerations

Diagnosis during pregnancy involves:

1. Reliance on clinical features to minimize invasive procedures
2. Careful consideration of the risk-benefit ratio of skin biopsy if needed
3. Differential diagnosis including pregnancy-specific dermatoses

9.2.3 Treatment Challenges

Managing JLI during pregnancy and lactation requires:

1. Careful selection of treatments that are safe for both mother and fetus/infant
2. Balancing the need for disease control with potential risks of medications
3. Consideration of the impact of untreated disease on maternal well-being

9.2.4 Safe Treatment Options

Preferred treatments during pregnancy and lactation include:

1. Topical corticosteroids (low to medium potency), used sparingly
2. Topical calcineurin inhibitors, with caution
3. Antihistamines for symptomatic relief, selecting those with established safety profiles
4. Non-pharmacological approaches, including meticulous sun protection

9.2.5 Treatments to Avoid

Certain treatments should be avoided or used with extreme caution:

1. Systemic corticosteroids, except when absolutely necessary
2. Antimalarials, due to potential risks to the fetus
3. Immunosuppressants like methotrexate, which are contraindicated in pregnancy
4. Phototherapy, particularly PUVA, due to potential risks

9.2.6 Postpartum and Lactation Considerations

Special considerations for the postpartum period include:

1. Potential for disease flare after delivery
2. Safety of treatments during breastfeeding
3. Need for contraception if using teratogenic medications postpartum

9.2.7 Case Study: JLI in Pregnancy

"Emma, a 30-year-old woman with a 5-year history of JLI, became pregnant. Her JLI initially improved during the first trimester but flared in the third trimester. Management focused on topical tacrolimus for facial lesions and careful sun avoidance. Postpartum, she experienced a significant flare, requiring a short course of low-dose prednisone while breastfeeding, under close monitoring."

9.3 Jessner's Lymphocytic Infiltrate in the Elderly

JLI in older adults presents unique challenges related to comorbidities, polypharmacy, and age-related changes in skin and immune function.

9.3.1 Clinical Presentation in the Elderly

JLI in older patients may present with:

1. More subtle clinical features due to age-related skin changes
2. Potential overlap with other age-related skin conditions
3. Increased likelihood of extensive or atypical distribution
4. Possible association with other autoimmune or inflammatory conditions more common in the elderly

9.3.2 Diagnostic Challenges

Diagnosing JLI in the elderly can be complicated by:

1. Presence of multiple dermatological conditions simultaneously
2. Age-related changes in skin that may alter typical histopathological features
3. Potential reluctance to undergo skin biopsy
4. Need to differentiate from cutaneous lymphoma, which is more common in this age group

9.3.3 Comorbidities and Their Impact

Common comorbidities in elderly patients with JLI may include:

1. Cardiovascular disease, affecting treatment choices
2. Diabetes, impacting wound healing and infection risk
3. Cognitive impairment, affecting treatment adherence and self-care
4. Polypharmacy, increasing the risk of drug interactions

9.3.4 Treatment Considerations

Managing JLI in the elderly requires attention to:

1. Potential drug interactions with existing medications
2. Altered pharmacokinetics and pharmacodynamics in older adults
3. Increased susceptibility to side effects of both topical and systemic treatments
4. Balancing disease control with overall quality of life and functional status

9.3.5 Tailored Treatment Approaches

Treatment strategies may include:

1. Preference for topical treatments to minimize systemic effects
2. Careful use of systemic therapies, with close monitoring for side effects
3. Consideration of the patient's ability to apply treatments independently
4. Emphasis on skin care and sun protection appropriate for aging skin

9.3.6 Psychosocial Aspects

Special attention should be paid to:

1. Impact of JLI on overall quality of life in the context of aging
2. Potential for social isolation due to visible skin condition
3. Need for support in managing treatment regimens
4. Consideration of the patient's living situation (e.g., independent, assisted living, nursing home)

9.3.7 Case Study: JLI in an Elderly Patient

"Mr. Johnson, an 78-year-old man with hypertension and type 2 diabetes, presented with a 2-year history of persistent erythematous plaques on his face and upper back. Biopsy confirmed JLI. Management included low-potency topical corticosteroids and sun protection. Adherence was improved by simplifying his skin care routine and involving his family in care coordination."

9.4 Jessner's Lymphocytic Infiltrate in Immunocompromised Patients

Immunocompromised individuals with JLI require special consideration due to their altered immune status and increased vulnerability to complications.

9.4.1 Causes of Immunocompromise

Common causes in JLI patients may include:

1. HIV/AIDS
2. Organ transplantation and associated immunosuppressive therapy
3. Hematological malignancies
4. Chronic use of immunosuppressive medications for other conditions

9.4.2 Clinical Presentation

JLI in immunocompromised patients may present with:

1. More extensive or severe cutaneous involvement
2. Atypical clinical features or distribution
3. Increased risk of secondary infections
4. Potential for more rapid progression or treatment resistance

9.4.3 Diagnostic Challenges

Diagnosis in this population is complicated by:

1. Broader differential diagnosis, including opportunistic infections and malignancies
2. Potential for atypical histopathological features due to altered immune responses
3. Need for more extensive workup to exclude other conditions
4. Importance of considering JLI as a potential marker of immune reconstitution in HIV patients starting antiretroviral therapy

9.4.4 Treatment Considerations

Managing JLI in immunocompromised patients requires:

1. Careful balance between controlling JLI and avoiding further immuno-suppression
2. Increased vigilance for infections and other complications
3. Consideration of potential interactions with other medications
4. Close collaboration between dermatologists and other specialists (e.g., infectious disease, oncology, transplant medicine)

9.4.5 Tailored Treatment Approaches

Treatment strategies may include:

1. Preference for topical treatments where possible
2. Cautious use of systemic immunosuppressants, weighing risks and benefits carefully
3. Consideration of antimicrobial prophylaxis in some cases
4. Emphasis on skin care and infection prevention

9.4.6 Monitoring and Follow-up

Special considerations for follow-up include:

1. More frequent monitoring for disease progression and complications
2. Regular skin examinations to detect potential malignancies
3. Coordination of care with other medical teams involved in the patient's management
4. Education on signs of infection or other complications requiring prompt medical attention

9.4.7 Case Study: JLI in an Immunocompromised Patient

"Lisa, a 45-year-old woman with a history of kidney transplantation 3 years ago, developed multiple erythematous plaques on her face and upper trunk. Biopsy confirmed JLI, but also raised concern for potential post-transplant lymphoproliferative disorder. Management involved careful tapering of her transplant immunosuppression, use of topical tacrolimus, and close monitoring in collaboration with her transplant team."

9.5 Jessner's Lymphocytic Infiltrate in Patients with Autoimmune Comorbidities

The co-existence of JLI with other autoimmune conditions presents unique diagnostic and management challenges.

9.5.1 Common Autoimmune Associations

JLI may be associated with various autoimmune conditions, including:

1. Systemic lupus erythematosus
2. Sjögren's syndrome
3. Rheumatoid arthritis
4. Autoimmune thyroid diseases

9.5.2 Diagnostic Complexities

Diagnosis in this context is complicated by:

1. Overlap in clinical features between JLI and cutaneous manifestations of other autoimmune diseases
2. Potential for JLI to be a cutaneous marker of systemic autoimmune disease
3. Need for comprehensive autoimmune workup in JLI patients
4. Challenges in distinguishing JLI from lupus erythematosus tumidus

9.5.3 Treatment Challenges

Managing JLI in patients with autoimmune comorbidities involves:

1. Coordinating treatment with management of the coexisting autoimmune condition

2. Balancing the use of immunomodulatory therapies
3. Monitoring for progression or development of additional autoimmune manifestations
4. Considering the impact of treatments on multiple conditions simultaneously

9.5.4 Tailored Management Strategies

Approaches may include:

1. Use of systemic therapies that can address both JLI and the coexisting autoimmune condition (e.g., hydroxychloroquine)
2. Careful selection of topical treatments to avoid exacerbating other cutaneous autoimmune manifestations
3. Emphasis on lifestyle modifications and sun protection, which may benefit multiple conditions
4. Regular screening for development of additional autoimmune conditions

9.5.5 Multidisciplinary Care

Effective management often requires:

1. Close collaboration between dermatologists and rheumatologists
2. Regular communication among all healthcare providers involved in the patient's care
3. Comprehensive patient education on managing multiple autoimmune conditions
4. Consideration of the cumulative impact of multiple conditions on quality of life

9.5.6 Case Study: JLI with Autoimmune Comorbidity

"Maria, a 50-year-old woman with Sjögren's syndrome, developed persistent erythematous plaques on her cheeks and upper chest. Biopsy confirmed JLI, but serologic workup also revealed positive ANA and anti-Ro antibodies. Management involved hydroxychloroquine, which addressed both her Sjögren's symptoms and JLI, along with topical tacrolimus for persistent facial lesions."

9.6 Jessner's Lymphocytic Infiltrate in Skin of Color

JLI presenting in patients with darker skin tones requires special consideration in diagnosis and management.

9.6.1 Clinical Presentation

In skin of color, JLI may present with:

1. Less apparent erythema, making lesions more subtle
2. Greater tendency for hyperpigmentation or hypopigmentation
3. Potential for more prominent textural changes
4. Increased risk of post-inflammatory pigmentary alterations

9.6.2 Diagnostic Challenges

Diagnosing JLI in skin of color involves:

1. Higher index of suspicion due to less obvious clinical features
2. Need for careful examination under good lighting conditions
3. Potential use of dermoscopy to enhance visualization of subtle features
4. Importance of biopsy for definitive diagnosis, with awareness of potential for pigmentary changes at biopsy sites

9.6.3 Treatment Considerations

Management strategies should consider:

1. Increased risk of post-inflammatory hyperpigmentation with certain treatments
2. Potential for hypopigmentation with overly aggressive topical steroid use
3. Careful selection of phototherapy protocols to minimize pigmentary changes
4. Use of treatments that address both inflammation and pigmentary alterations

9.6.4 Patient Education

Special emphasis should be placed on:

1. Importance of sun protection to prevent worsening of pigmentary changes
2. Realistic expectations regarding treatment outcomes and timeline
3. Proper use of cosmetic camouflage techniques if desired
4. Recognition of signs indicating need for medical re-evaluation

9.6.5 Case Study: JLI in Skin of Color

"Aisha, a 35-year-old woman with Fitzpatrick skin type V, presented with a 1-year history of hyperpigmented plaques on her cheeks, initially misdiagnosed as melasma. Biopsy confirmed JLI. Management included topical tacrolimus, careful sun protection, and short courses of low-potency topical steroids for flares, with emphasis on preventing post-inflammatory hyperpigmentation."

Conclusion

Jessner's Lymphocytic Infiltrate in special populations presents unique challenges that require tailored approaches to diagnosis, management, and patient care. Whether dealing with pediatric cases, pregnant patients, the elderly, immunocompromised individuals, those with autoimmune comorbidities, or patients with skin of color, healthcare providers must adapt their strategies to address the specific needs and risks of each group.

Key principles in managing JLI in these special populations include:

1. Maintaining a high index of suspicion for atypical presentations
2. Carefully weighing the risks and benefits of diagnostic procedures and treatments
3. Adapting treatment plans to account for age-related factors, comorbidities, and potential drug interactions
4. Emphasizing interdisciplinary collaboration to provide comprehensive care
5. Providing patient education tailored to the specific needs and challenges of each group

By recognizing and addressing the unique aspects of JLI in these special populations, healthcare providers can optimize outcomes and improve quality of life for all patients living with this challenging condition. As research in this area continues to

CHAPTER 10

Research Frontiers and Future Directions in Jessner's Lymphocytic Infiltrate

As our understanding of Jessner's Lymphocytic Infiltrate (JLI) continues to evolve, new avenues of research are constantly emerging. This chapter explores the cutting-edge research in JLI, ongoing clinical trials, and potential future directions that may revolutionize our approach to diagnosing, treating, and managing this condition.

10.1 Advances in Understanding JLI Pathogenesis

Recent years have seen significant progress in unraveling the underlying mechanisms of JLI.

10.1.1 Immunological Insights

Emerging research focuses on:

1. Characterization of the T cell subsets involved in JLI lesions
2. Role of innate immune responses in initiating and perpetuating inflammation
3. Potential involvement of B cells and humoral immunity
4. Cytokine and chemokine profiles specific to JLI

10.1.2 Genetic Studies

Ongoing genetic investigations include:

1. Genome-wide association studies (GWAS) to identify susceptibility loci
2. Exploration of epigenetic modifications in JLI
3. Investigation of familial cases to understand hereditary components
4. Pharmacogenomic studies to predict treatment responses

10.1.3 Environmental Triggers

Research into environmental factors involves:

1. Examination of the role of UV radiation in JLI pathogenesis
2. Investigation of potential infectious triggers, including viral associations
3. Exploration of occupational and lifestyle factors that may influence JLI development

10.1.4 Microbiome Studies

Emerging microbiome research in JLI includes:

1. Characterization of skin microbiome alterations in JLI lesions
2. Investigation of the gut-skin axis in JLI pathogenesis
3. Exploration of microbiome-based therapeutic approaches

10.2 Advances in Diagnostic Techniques

New diagnostic approaches are being developed to enhance accuracy and ease of JLI diagnosis.

10.2.1 Non-invasive Imaging Techniques

Promising technologies include:

1. High-resolution optical coherence tomography (OCT) for in vivo visualization of skin structures
2. Reflectance confocal microscopy for cellular-level imaging of JLI lesions
3. Multiphoton microscopy for detailed assessment of collagen and elastin changes

10.2.2 Biomarker Discovery

Ongoing research focuses on identifying:

1. Serum biomarkers for JLI diagnosis and disease activity monitoring
2. Tissue biomarkers to differentiate JLI from other lymphocytic infiltrates
3. Genetic markers predictive of disease course or treatment response

10.2.3 Artificial Intelligence in Diagnosis

Emerging applications of AI include:

1. Machine learning algorithms for analyzing clinical images of JLI
2. AI-assisted interpretation of histopathological slides
3. Development of decision support tools for JLI diagnosis and management

10.3 Emerging Therapeutic Approaches

Novel treatment strategies are being explored to improve outcomes in JLI.

10.3.1 Targeted Immunotherapies

Promising areas of investigation include:

1. JAK inhibitors for modulating T cell-mediated inflammation
2. IL-23/IL-17 axis inhibitors, building on success in other inflammatory skin conditions
3. Targeted depletion of specific T cell subsets involved in JLI pathogenesis

10.3.2 Biologics

Ongoing research on biologics focuses on:

1. Anti-TNF agents for refractory JLI cases
2. B cell-targeted therapies, exploring the role of B cells in JLI
3. Costimulation blockade agents to modulate T cell activation

10.3.3 Small Molecule Inhibitors

Investigation of small molecule drugs includes:

1. Tyrosine kinase inhibitors for modulating intracellular signaling pathways
2. Phosphodiesterase inhibitors for their anti-inflammatory properties
3. Proteasome inhibitors, exploring their potential in immune modulation

10.3.4 Photodynamic Therapy

Advances in photodynamic therapy (PDT) for JLI involve:

1. Development of new photosensitizers with improved efficacy and safety profiles
2. Optimization of light sources and treatment protocols for JLI
3. Combination approaches integrating PDT with other treatment modalities

10.3.5 Nanotechnology-based Treatments

Emerging nanotechnology applications include:

1. Nanoparticle-based drug delivery systems for enhanced topical treatments
2. Nanoengineered materials for controlled release of anti-inflammatory agents
3. Photothermal therapy using nanoparticles activated by near-infrared light

10.4 Ongoing Clinical Trials

Several clinical trials are currently underway, exploring new treatments and management strategies for JLI.

10.4.1 Phase I Trials

Early-stage trials are investigating:

1. Safety and tolerability of novel JAK inhibitors in JLI

2. Dose-finding studies for repurposed drugs showing promise in JLI
3. First-in-human studies of innovative targeted therapies

10.4.2 Phase II Trials

Mid-stage trials are focusing on:

1. Efficacy of IL-23 inhibitors in moderate to severe JLI
2. Comparative studies of different phototherapy protocols
3. Evaluation of combination therapies for refractory JLI

10.4.3 Phase III Trials

Late-stage trials include:

1. Large-scale studies on the long-term efficacy and safety of systemic treatments
2. Comparative effectiveness trials of established and newer therapies
3. Quality of life outcomes with various treatment approaches

10.4.4 Other Clinical Studies

Additional ongoing research includes:

1. Observational studies on the natural history of JLI
2. Patient registry initiatives to collect long-term data on JLI outcomes
3. Pharmacoeconomic studies evaluating cost-effectiveness of different treatments

10.5 Personalized Medicine in JLI

The future of JLI management lies in personalized approaches tailored to individual patients.

10.5.1 Genetic Profiling

Advances in genetic analysis aim to:

1. Identify genetic markers predictive of disease severity and progression
2. Develop genetic tests to guide treatment selection
3. Explore gene therapy approaches for JLI

10.5.2 Immunophenotyping

Detailed immune profiling seeks to:

1. Characterize individual patients' immune signatures
2. Match specific immune profiles with optimal treatment strategies
3. Monitor immune responses to guide treatment adjustments

10.5.3 Precision Medicine Algorithms

Development of decision support tools includes:

1. Integration of clinical, genetic, and immunological data to guide treatment decisions
2. Machine learning models for predicting treatment outcomes
3. Personalized risk stratification for JLI complications

10.6 Technological Innovations in JLI Management

Emerging technologies are poised to transform JLI care.

10.6.1 Telemedicine and Remote Monitoring

Advancements include:

1. Development of smartphone-based apps for tracking JLI symptoms and treatment response
2. Teledermatology platforms for remote consultation and follow-up
3. Wearable devices for continuous monitoring of environmental triggers and physiological responses

10.6.2 Virtual and Augmented Reality

Potential applications encompass:

1. VR-based tools for patient education about JLI
2. AR applications to assist in precise topical treatment application
3. VR environments for psychological support and stress reduction

10.6.3 3D Printing in JLI Care

Innovative uses of 3D printing technology include:

1. Customized wound dressings for JLI lesions
2. Patient-specific models for surgical planning in complex cases
3. 3D-printed drug delivery systems for controlled release of medications

10.7 Psychodermatological Approaches

The integration of psychological and dermatological care continues to evolve.

10.7.1 Mind-Body Interventions

Ongoing research explores:

1. Effectiveness of mindfulness-based stress reduction in managing JLI flares
2. Impact of cognitive-behavioral therapy on treatment adherence and outcomes
3. Role of psychoneuroimmunology in JLI pathogenesis and management

10.7.2 Quality of Life Measures

Development of JLI-specific tools includes:

1. Validation of disease-specific quality of life questionnaires
2. Integration of patient-reported outcomes in clinical trials and routine care
3. Exploration of the economic and social impact of JLI

10.7.3 Psychodermatology Clinics

Expansion of specialized care lmodels involves:

1. Establishment of integrated psychodermatology clinics for JLI patients
2. Development of training programs for psychodermatology specialists
3. Evaluation of cost-effectiveness of integrated care approaches

10.8 Lifestyle and Complementary Approaches

Research into non-pharmacological interventions is gaining momentum.

10.8.1 Dietary Interventions

Nutritional studies focus on:

1. Impact of anti-inflammatory diets on JLI symptoms
2. Role of specific nutrients or dietary supplements in managing JLI
3. Gut microbiome modulation through dietary interventions

10.8.2 Exercise and Physical Activity

Investigations explore:

1. Effects of regular exercise on JLI disease activity
2. Optimal types and intensities of physical activity for JLI patients
3. Impact of exercise on quality of life and psychological well-being in JLI

10.8.3 Complementary and Alternative Medicine

Research into alternative approaches includes:

1. Efficacy of acupuncture in managing JLI symptoms
2. Potential benefits of herbal medicines in JLI treatment
3. Role of mind-body practices like yoga and tai chi in JLI management

10.9 Environmental and Occupational Health Research

Understanding environmental influences on JLI is a growing area of interest.

10.9.1 UV Radiation Studies

Ongoing research examines:

1. Molecular mechanisms of UV-induced exacerbation in JLI
2. Development of more effective photoprotection strategies
3. Potential therapeutic applications of controlled UV exposure

10.9.2 Occupational Exposures

Investigations focus on:

1. Identification of occupational risk factors for JLI development or exacerbation
2. Development of workplace interventions to reduce JLI risk
3. Long-term outcomes of occupational JLI cases

10.9.3 Climate Change Impact

Emerging research explores:

1. Effects of changing climate patterns on JLI prevalence and severity
2. Adaptation strategies for JLI patients in the context of global warming
3. Environmental health policies to mitigate climate-related impacts on JLI

10.10 Global Health Perspectives

Research is expanding to address JLI in diverse global contexts.

10.10.1 Epidemiological Studies

Global research initiatives aim to:

1. Determine worldwide prevalence and incidence of JLI
2. Identify geographic and ethnic variations in JLI presentation and outcomes
3. Explore socioeconomic factors influencing JLI care globally

10.10.2 Health Disparities Research

Investigations focus on:

1. Access to JLI diagnosis and treatment in resource-limited settings
2. Development of cost-effective management strategies for low-resource environments
3. Cultural factors influencing JLI perception and care-seeking behaviors

10.10.3 Global Collaborations

International research efforts include:

1. Establishment of global JLI patient registries
2. Multicenter clinical trials spanning diverse populations
3. Knowledge exchange programs to improve JLI care worldwide

10.11 Translational Research Initiatives

Bridging the gap between basic science and clinical application is a key focus.

10.11.1 Bioengineering Approaches

Innovative research includes:

1. Development of skin-on-a-chip models for JLI research
2. Bioengineered skin substitutes for studying JLI pathogenesis
3. Tissue engineering approaches for skin regeneration in JLI

10.11.2 Drug Repurposing

Ongoing efforts explore:

1. Screening of existing drug libraries for potential JLI treatments
2. Computational approaches to predict drug efficacy in JLI
3. Fast-track clinical trials of repurposed drugs showing promise in JLI

10.11.3 Biomarker Translation

Research aims to:

1. Validate laboratory biomarkers for clinical use in JLI
2. Develop point-of-care diagnostic tests for JLI
3. Integrate biomarker data into clinical decision-making algorithms

10.12 Future Challenges and Opportunities

As research in JLI progresses, several challenges and opportunities emerge.

10.12.1 Challenges

Key obstacles include:

1. Rarity of JLI, making large-scale clinical studies challenging
2. Heterogeneity of JLI presentation, complicating standardized approaches
3. Long-term safety concerns with novel immunomodulatory therapies
4. Balancing efficacy, safety, and cost in developing new treatments

10.12.2 Opportunities

Promising avenues include:

1. Leveraging big data and artificial intelligence for JLI research
2. Developing international collaborations to pool resources and knowledge
3. Exploring crossover findings from research in related autoimmune conditions
4. Engaging patient advocacy groups in setting research priorities

10.12.3 Ethical Considerations

Future research must address:

1. Ethical implications of genetic testing and personalized medicine in JLI
2. Ensuring equitable access to advanced therapies
3. Balancing innovation with patient safety in clinical trials
4. Addressing privacy concerns in the era of digital health and big data

Conclusion

The landscape of Jessner's Lymphocytic Infiltrate research is rapidly evolving, offering exciting prospects for improved understanding, diagnosis, and management of this challenging condition. From advances in basic science unraveling the pathogenesis of JLI to innovative clinical approaches and cutting-edge technologies, the future holds promise for significant improvements in patient care.

Key areas of future focus include:

1. Personalized medicine approaches tailored to individual patient profiles
2. Integration of advanced technologies in diagnosis and management
3. Development of targeted therapies based on improved understanding of JLI immunopathogenesis
4. Holistic approaches encompassing both physical and psychological aspects of JLI
5. Global initiatives to address JLI in diverse populations and settings

As research progresses, it is crucial to maintain a patient-centered approach, ensuring that advances in science and technology translate into meaningful improvements in quality of life for individuals living with JLI. Collaboration between researchers, clinicians, patients, and advocacy groups will be key to driving progress and overcoming the challenges that lie ahead.

The future of JLI research is bright, with the potential to transform our approach to this condition from diagnosis through long-term management. As we look forward, the hope is that continued research and innovation will lead to more effective, personalized, and accessible care for all patients affected by Jessner's Lymphocytic Infiltrate.

CHAPTER 11

Holistic Approaches and Complementary Therapies

While conventional medical treatments form the cornerstone of managing Jessner's Lymphocytic Infiltrate (JLI), many patients seek complementary approaches to enhance their overall well-being and potentially improve their condition. This chapter explores various holistic and complementary therapies that may be beneficial for individuals with JLI, discussing their potential benefits, limitations, and integration with standard medical care.

11.1 The Role of Holistic Medicine in JLI Management

Holistic medicine approaches JLI as part of the whole person, considering physical, emotional, social, and spiritual aspects of health.

11.1.1 Principles of Holistic Care in JLI

Key concepts include:

1. Treating the person, not just the disease
2. Emphasizing the body's innate healing abilities
3. Considering the interconnectedness of body systems
4. Focusing on prevention and wellness alongside treatment

11.1.2 Benefits of a Holistic Approach

Potential advantages include:

1. Addressing multiple aspects of patient well-being
2. Empowering patients to take an active role in their health
3. Potentially reducing reliance on pharmacological interventions
4. Improving overall quality of life beyond skin symptoms

11.1.3 Challenges and Considerations

Important factors to consider:

1. Variability in evidence base for different holistic approaches
2. Potential interactions with conventional treatments
3. Need for open communication between patients and healthcare providers about all therapies used

11.2 Diet and Nutrition in JLI Management

While direct dietary links to JLI are not well-established, nutrition can play a role in overall skin health and inflammation management.

11.2.1 Anti-Inflammatory Diets

Potential benefits of anti-inflammatory eating patterns:

1. Mediterranean diet: Rich in omega-3 fatty acids, antioxidants, and fiber
2. Plant-based diets: High in phytonutrients with anti-inflammatory properties
3. Low glycemic index diets: May help reduce inflammation and oxidative

stress

11.2.2 Specific Nutrients of Interest

Nutrients that may support skin health include:

1. Omega-3 fatty acids: Found in fish, flaxseed, and walnuts
2. Antioxidants: Including vitamins C, E, and beta-carotene
3. Zinc: Important for skin healing and immune function
4. Vitamin D: Often low in JLI patients, particularly those avoiding sun exposure

11.2.3 Food Sensitivities and Elimination Diets

Considerations for identifying potential dietary triggers:

1. Keeping a food diary to track potential correlations with flares
2. Supervised elimination diets to identify possible food sensitivities
3. Gradual reintroduction of foods to confirm any associations

11.2.4 Hydration and Skin Health

The importance of adequate hydration:

1. Role of proper hydration in maintaining skin barrier function
2. Potential benefits of herbal teas with anti-inflammatory properties
3. Consideration of electrolyte balance, particularly in hot climates or with increased sweating

11.3 Mind-Body Techniques

Mind-body practices can help manage stress, which may influence JLI flares and overall well-being.

11.3.1 Mindfulness and Meditation

Potential benefits for JLI patients:

1. Stress reduction, which may help manage flares
2. Improved coping with chronic illness
3. Enhanced overall well-being and quality of life

Specific techniques:

1. Mindfulness-Based Stress Reduction (MBSR)
2. Transcendental Meditation
3. Guided imagery focused on skin healing

11.3.2 Yoga and Tai Chi

These practices may offer:

1. Gentle exercise suitable for most fitness levels
2. Stress reduction and improved body awareness
3. Potential immune-modulating effects through mind-body connection

11.3.3 Biofeedback

Applications in JLI management:

1. Learning to control physiological processes that may influence skin inflammation
2. Stress management techniques using real-time feedback
3. Potential for reducing symptomatic discomfort associated with JLI lesions

11.3.4 Cognitive Behavioral Therapy (CBT)

While primarily a psychological intervention, CBT has mind-body components:

1. Addressing negative thought patterns related to skin appearance
2. Developing coping strategies for managing chronic illness
3. Techniques for managing stress and anxiety related to JLI

11.4 Herbal Medicine and Natural Remedies

Various herbal and natural remedies have been explored for their potential benefits in skin health and inflammation management.

11.4.1 Topical Herbal Preparations

Herbs with potential anti-inflammatory properties:

1. Aloe vera: Soothing and potentially anti-inflammatory
2. Chamomile: May have calming effects on irritated skin
3. Calendula: Traditional use for skin healing and inflammation
4. Green tea: Rich in antioxidants with potential anti-inflammatory effects

11.4.2 Oral Herbal Supplements

Herbs that may support skin health and immune function:

1. Turmeric: Contains curcumin, known for anti-inflammatory properties
2. Ginger: May have immune-modulating effects
3. Boswellia: Traditional use in managing inflammatory conditions
4. Milk thistle: Potential liver-supportive properties, which may indirectly benefit skin health

11.4.3 Essential Oils

Potential applications in JLI management:

1. Lavender oil: May have calming and anti-inflammatory properties
2. Tea tree oil: Known for its antimicrobial effects
3. Frankincense oil: Traditional use in skin health and inflammation
4. Considerations for safe use, including proper dilution and patch testing

11.4.4 Cautions and Considerations

Important factors when considering herbal remedies:

1. Potential interactions with conventional medications
2. Variability in product quality and standardization
3. Importance of informing healthcare providers about all supplements used
4. Need for further research to establish efficacy and safety in JLI

11.5 Acupuncture and Traditional Chinese Medicine

Traditional Chinese Medicine (TCM) offers a holistic approach that may complement conventional JLI management.

11.5.1 Principles of TCM in Skin Health

Key concepts in TCM approach to skin disorders:

1. Balance of Yin and Yang energies
2. Regulation of Qi (vital energy) flow
3. Addressing underlying imbalances in organ systems

11.5.2 Acupuncture for JLI

Potential benefits and considerations:

1. Possible immune-modulating effects
2. Stress reduction and overall well-being
3. Consideration of acupuncture points traditionally associated with skin health
4. Importance of treatment by qualified practitioners

11.5.3 Chinese Herbal Medicine

Approaches in TCM herbal therapy:

1. Customized herbal formulations based on individual diagnosis
2. Potential use of herbs with cooling or detoxifying properties for skin inflammation
3. Consideration of overall constitution and not just skin symptoms
4. Need for caution regarding potential herb-drug interactions

11.5.4 Other TCM Modalities

Additional techniques that may be employed:

1. Cupping: Potential for improving local circulation
2. Gua sha: Traditional scraping technique, used cautiously in skin conditions
3. Moxibustion: Warming therapy, used judiciously in inflammatory conditions

11.6 Physical Therapies and Bodywork

Various physical therapies may offer benefits for overall well-being and potentially for skin health.

11.6.1 Massage Therapy

Potential benefits and considerations:

1. Stress reduction and relaxation
2. Improved circulation, which may support skin health
3. Lymphatic drainage techniques for potential immune support
4. Cautions regarding pressure and techniques over active JLI lesions

11.6.2 Hydrotherapy

Water-based therapies that may be beneficial:

1. Balneotherapy: Bathing in mineral-rich waters
2. Contrast hydrotherapy: Alternating hot and cold applications for circulation

3. Gentle aquatic exercises for overall health
4. Consideration of water quality and temperature for sensitive skin

11.6.3 Reflexology

Potential applications in JLI management:

1. Stress reduction through foot or hand manipulation
2. Traditional associations of specific reflex points with skin health
3. General relaxation and well-being support

11.6.4 Chiropractic and Osteopathic Approaches

Considerations for manual therapies:

1. Potential benefits for overall health and well-being
2. Addressing musculoskeletal issues that may indirectly affect stress and skin health
3. Caution with manipulations over areas of active JLI lesions

11.7 Energy Healing and Biofield Therapies

While controversial and lacking strong scientific evidence, some patients find value in energy-based approaches.

11.7.1 Reiki

Principles and potential benefits:

1. Hands-on or distant energy healing technique

2. Aimed at promoting relaxation and overall well-being
3. Consideration as a complementary relaxation technique

11.7.2 Therapeutic Touch

Concepts and applications:

1. Energy-based practice developed by nurses
2. Focused on balancing the body's energy field
3. Potential stress-reduction benefits

11.7.3 Electromagnetic Therapies

Emerging areas of investigation:

1. Pulsed electromagnetic field therapy: Potential anti-inflammatory effects
2. Low-level light therapy: Possible benefits for skin health
3. Need for further research to establish efficacy and safety in JLI

11.8 Stress Management and Lifestyle Modifications

Comprehensive lifestyle approaches can support overall health and potentially influence JLI management.

11.8.1 Sleep Optimization

Importance of quality sleep:

1. Role of sleep in immune function and skin repair

2. Strategies for improving sleep hygiene
3. Consideration of circadian rhythms in skin health

11.8.2 Exercise and Physical Activity

Benefits of regular exercise:

1. Stress reduction and mood improvement
2. Potential immune-modulating effects
3. Improved overall health and well-being
4. Considerations for exercise intensity and sweating with active JLI lesions

11.8.3 Stress Reduction Techniques

Additional approaches for managing stress:

1. Time management and prioritization strategies
2. Hobby engagement for relaxation and fulfillment
3. Social support and community involvement
4. Nature exposure and eco-therapy

11.8.4 Environmental Considerations

Addressing potential environmental triggers:

1. Optimizing indoor air quality
2. Choosing skin-friendly fabrics and detergents
3. Minimizing exposure to potential irritants or allergens
4. Creating a healing home environment

11.9 Nutritional Supplements

While diet should be the primary source of nutrients, some supplements may be considered.

11.9.1 Omega-3 Fatty Acids

Potential benefits and sources:

1. Anti-inflammatory properties
2. Fish oil or algae-based supplements for those avoiding fish
3. Consideration of appropriate dosage and quality

11.9.2 Probiotics and Prebiotics

Potential role in skin health:

1. Modulation of gut microbiome, which may influence skin health
2. Specific strains that may have immune-modulating effects
3. Importance of choosing quality supplements with research support

11.9.3 Antioxidants

Supplements that may support skin health:

1. Vitamin C: Important for collagen synthesis and antioxidant defense
2. Vitamin E: Fat-soluble antioxidant that may support skin barrier function
3. Coenzyme Q10: Potential benefits for cellular energy production in skin

11.9.4 Vitamin D

Considerations for supplementation:

1. Common deficiency, especially in those avoiding sun exposure
2. Potential immune-modulating effects
3. Importance of monitoring blood levels for appropriate dosing

11.10 Integrating Complementary Approaches with Conventional Care

Successfully incorporating holistic and complementary therapies requires careful consideration and communication.

11.10.1 Communication with Healthcare Providers

Importance of open dialogue:

1. Informing dermatologists and other providers about all therapies used
2. Discussing potential interactions or contraindications
3. Seeking guidance on integrating complementary approaches

11.10.2 Developing an Integrated Care Plan

Strategies for comprehensive care:

1. Prioritizing therapies based on evidence and individual needs
2. Establishing clear goals and metrics for evaluating complementary approaches
3. Regular reassessment and adjustment of the integrated care plan

11.10.3 Patient Education and Empowerment

Supporting informed decision-making:

1. Providing reliable resources on complementary therapies
2. Encouraging critical evaluation of claims and evidence
3. Empowering patients to be active participants in their care

11.10.4 Monitoring and Safety Considerations

Ensuring safe integration of therapies:

1. Tracking potential interactions between complementary and conventional treatments
2. Monitoring for adverse effects or unexpected changes in JLI symptoms
3. Establishing clear guidelines for when to seek medical evaluation

11.11 Future Directions in Holistic JLI Management

As interest in holistic approaches grows, several areas warrant further exploration.

11.11.1 Research Needs

Priorities for advancing understanding:

1. Well-designed clinical trials on complementary therapies for JLI
2. Investigation of potential mechanisms of action for promising approaches
3. Long-term studies on the safety and efficacy of integrated care models

11.11.2 Personalized Holistic Approaches

Tailoring therapies to individual needs:

1. Consideration of genetic, environmental, and lifestyle factors
2. Developing personalized protocols combining conventional and complementary approaches
3. Leveraging technology for tracking and optimizing individualized care plans

11.11.3 Integration into Standard Care Models

Opportunities for broader implementation:

1. Incorporating holistic assessments into routine JLI care
2. Developing training programs for healthcare providers on integrative approaches
3. Exploring cost-effectiveness and potential healthcare savings of comprehensive care models

Conclusion

Holistic and complementary approaches offer potential benefits for individuals living with Jessner's Lymphocytic Infiltrate, addressing not only skin symptoms but overall health and well-being. While many of these therapies require further research to establish their efficacy and safety specifically for JLI, they may provide valuable support when integrated thoughtfully with conventional medical care.

Key takeaways from this exploration of holistic approaches include:

1. The importance of a whole-person approach to JLI management
2. Potential benefits of dietary modifications, stress reduction techniques, and mind-body practices
3. The need for careful consideration and professional guidance when exploring herbal or supplement-based therapies
4. The value of open communication between patients and healthcare providers about all therapies used
5. The potential for personalized, integrated care plans that combine the best of conventional and complementary approaches

As research in this area continues to evolve, the hope is that a more comprehensive, evidence-based approach to JLI management will emerge, offering patients a wider range of options for improving their skin health and overall quality of life. While complementary therapies should not replace conventional medical treatments for JLI, they may offer valuable adjunctive support, empowering patients to take an active role in their health and well-being.

CHAPTER 12

Global Perspectives and Resources

Jessner's Lymphocytic Infiltrate (JLI) is a condition that affects individuals worldwide, yet its presentation, management, and impact can vary significantly across different cultural, geographical, and healthcare contexts. This chapter explores the global landscape of JLI, discussing international variations in approach, challenges in resource-limited settings, and the wealth of resources available to patients and healthcare providers around the world.

12.1 Epidemiology of JLI: A Global View

Understanding the worldwide prevalence and distribution of JLI is crucial for developing global strategies for its management.

12.1.1 Prevalence Across Regions

Current knowledge of JLI distribution:

1. Variations in reported prevalence across different countries and continents
2. Challenges in obtaining accurate global data due to potential under-diagnosis or misdiagnosis
3. Apparent higher prevalence in certain ethnic groups, though this may

be influenced by reporting biases

12.1.2 Factors Influencing Global Epidemiology

Considerations in interpreting global JLI data:

1. Genetic factors that may influence susceptibility in different populations
2. Environmental factors, including UV exposure patterns in different geographical areas
3. Variations in healthcare access and diagnostic capabilities across regions

12.1.3 Global Trends and Emerging Patterns

Observations on changing JLI epidemiology:

1. Potential increases in diagnosis rates with improved awareness and diagnostic capabilities
2. Emerging data on JLI in previously understudied populations
3. Impact of global migration patterns on JLI distribution and management

12.2 Cultural Perspectives on Skin Conditions

The perception and impact of JLI can vary significantly across different cultural contexts.

12.2.1 Cultural Attitudes Towards Skin Appearance

Variations in the social impact of visible skin conditions:

1. Cultures with high emphasis on "perfect" skin and potential stigma of skin disorders
2. Societies where skin markings may have different cultural significance
3. Impact of cultural beauty standards on the psychological burden of JLI

12.2.2 Traditional Healing Practices

Integration of cultural healing traditions:

1. Use of traditional herbal remedies for skin conditions in various cultures
2. Role of traditional healers in managing skin disorders in some societies
3. Challenges and opportunities in integrating traditional practices with modern medicine

12.2.3 Religion and Spirituality in JLI Management

Influence of spiritual beliefs on coping and treatment:

1. Religious perspectives on health and illness that may affect JLI management
2. Use of prayer or spiritual practices as complementary approaches
3. Considerations for healthcare providers in addressing spiritual aspects of care

12.3 Healthcare Systems and JLI Management

The approach to JLI can vary significantly depending on the structure and resources of different healthcare systems.

12.3.1 Variations in Healthcare Delivery Models

Impact of different systems on JLI care:

1. Universal healthcare systems and access to dermatological services
2. Private healthcare models and potential disparities in access to specialized care
3. Hybrid systems and their impact on continuity of care for chronic conditions like JLI

12.3.2 Specialist Availability and Training

Global variations in dermatology resources:

1. Disparities in the number of trained dermatologists across different countries
2. Role of general practitioners in managing JLI in areas with limited specialist access
3. International training initiatives to improve dermatological care globally

12.3.3 Treatment Availability and Cost

Factors affecting access to JLI treatments worldwide:

1. Variations in drug availability and approval across different countries
2. Cost considerations and insurance coverage for JLI treatments in various systems
3. Impact of healthcare policies on access to newer or more expensive therapies

12.4 International Research Collaborations

Global cooperation is crucial for advancing our understanding and management of JLI.

12.4.1 Multinational Clinical Trials

Efforts to conduct large-scale studies:

1. Challenges in coordinating trials across different regulatory environments
2. Benefits of diverse patient populations in understanding JLI variability
3. Examples of successful international collaborations in JLI research

12.4.2 Data Sharing Initiatives

Global efforts to pool JLI data:

1. International registries for rare dermatological conditions including JLI
2. Challenges in standardizing data collection across different healthcare systems
3. Potential insights from big data approaches to global JLI information

12.4.3 International Research Networks

Collaborative structures advancing JLI knowledge:

1. Global dermatology research networks focusing on inflammatory skin conditions
2. Virtual collaboration platforms facilitating international knowledge

exchange

3. Role of international dermatology organizations in fostering research partnerships

12.5 Telemedicine and Global JLI Care

The rise of telemedicine offers new opportunities for global JLI management.

12.5.1 Teledermatology for JLI

Applications of remote dermatology services:

1. Use of store-and-forward systems for JLI diagnosis in remote areas
2. Live video consultations for follow-up and management
3. Challenges in accurately assessing JLI lesions via telemedicine

12.5.2 Mobile Health (mHealth) Applications

Smartphone-based tools for JLI care:

1. Apps for tracking JLI symptoms and treatment responses
2. Patient education platforms providing global access to JLI information
3. Potential for AI-assisted diagnosis using smartphone images

12.5.3 Global E-Learning Platforms

Online resources for healthcare provider education:

1. Webinars and virtual conferences on JLI management
2. Online courses and certifications in dermatology for global practition-

ers

3. Virtual case discussions facilitating global knowledge sharing

12.6 Challenges in Resource-Limited Settings

Managing JLI in areas with limited healthcare resources presents unique challenges.

12.6.1 Diagnostic Challenges

Obstacles in accurately identifying JLI:

1. Limited access to dermatopathology services for definitive diagnosis
2. Reliance on clinical diagnosis in the absence of biopsy capabilities
3. Strategies for improving diagnostic accuracy with limited resources

12.6.2 Treatment Availability

Addressing limitations in therapeutic options:

1. Focus on cost-effective treatments that are widely available
2. Strategies for adapting treatment protocols to available resources
3. Role of non-governmental organizations in improving access to treatments

12.6.3 Patient Education and Follow-up

Ensuring continuity of care in challenging settings:

1. Developing culturally appropriate patient education materials

2. Strategies for maintaining long-term follow-up in transient populations
3. Leveraging community health workers for ongoing JLI management

12.7 International Guidelines and Standards of Care

Efforts to standardize JLI management globally while accounting for regional variations.

12.7.1 International Consensus Statements

Development of globally applicable guidance:

1. Collaborative efforts to create international JLI management guidelines
2. Challenges in adapting recommendations to diverse healthcare contexts
3. Regular updates to incorporate new global research findings

12.7.2 Regional Adaptations

Tailoring guidelines to specific contexts:

1. Consideration of local resources, cultural factors, and healthcare systems
2. Region-specific treatment algorithms based on available therapies
3. Incorporation of traditional practices where appropriate and evidence-based

12.7.3 Quality Metrics and Outcome Measures

Standardizing assessment of JLI care quality:

1. Development of internationally recognized outcome measures for JLI
2. Challenges in implementing uniform quality metrics across diverse settings
3. Use of patient-reported outcomes to capture global patient experiences

12.8 Patient Advocacy and Support on a Global Scale

The role of international patient organizations in supporting the global JLI community.

12.8.1 International Patient Organizations

Global networks supporting JLI patients:

1. Examples of successful international JLI patient advocacy groups
2. Challenges in coordinating patient support across different cultures and languages
3. Role of patient organizations in driving global research agendas

12.8.2 Online Support Communities

Virtual platforms connecting JLI patients worldwide:

1. International online forums and support groups
2. Social media networks facilitating global patient connections
3. Considerations for ensuring accurate information sharing in online communities

12.8.3 Global Awareness Initiatives

Efforts to increase worldwide recognition of JLI:

1. International JLI awareness days or campaigns
2. Collaborations with broader dermatology awareness initiatives
3. Strategies for raising JLI awareness in regions with limited resources

12.9 Educational Resources for Patients and Providers

A wealth of information is available to support JLI understanding and management globally.

12.9.1 Multilingual Patient Education Materials

Resources for diverse patient populations:

1. Translated informational brochures and websites on JLI
2. Culturally adapted educational videos and animations
3. Pictorial guides for use in areas with low literacy rates

12.9.2 Professional Development Resources

Tools for healthcare provider education:

1. International dermatology textbooks and journals covering JLI
2. Online continuing medical education modules on JLI management
3. International fellowship programs for specialized training in cutaneous lymphocytic disorders

12.9.3 Global Health Education Initiatives

Efforts to improve worldwide dermatology knowledge:

1. Integration of JLI into global health dermatology curricula
2. Volunteer programs sending dermatology experts to resource-limited areas
3. Twinning programs pairing dermatology departments in different countries for knowledge exchange

12.10 Economic Impact of JLI: A Global Perspective

Understanding the worldwide economic burden of JLI is crucial for healthcare planning and resource allocation.

12.10.1 Direct Healthcare Costs

Variations in JLI-related expenses globally:

1. Differences in diagnostic and treatment costs across healthcare systems
2. Impact of medication pricing and availability on overall management costs
3. Long-term economic burden of chronic JLI care in different economies

12.10.2 Indirect Costs and Productivity Loss

Broader economic implications of JLI:

1. Global variations in work absenteeism and presenteeism due to JLI
2. Impact on career progression and earning potential across different societies
3. Societal costs related to psychological burden and quality of life impairment

12.10.3 Cost-Effectiveness Analyses

Evaluating the value of JLI interventions globally:

1. Challenges in conducting international cost-effectiveness studies
2. Variations in what is considered "cost-effective" across different economies
3. Impact of cost-effectiveness data on global treatment guidelines and policies

12.11 Environmental Factors and Global JLI Patterns

Exploring how global environmental variations may influence JLI presentation and management.

12.11.1 Climate and UV Exposure

Impact of geographical variations:

1. Differences in JLI presentation and course in tropical vs. temperate climates
2. Strategies for UV protection in different global environments
3. Potential impacts of climate change on future JLI patterns

12.11.2 Pollution and Industrial Exposures

Consideration of environmental triggers:

1. Potential role of air pollution in JLI exacerbation in different regions
2. Occupational exposures and JLI risk in various global industries
3. Environmental health policies and their impact on JLI management

12.11.3 Lifestyle and Dietary Factors

Global variations in potential JLI influences:

1. Differences in dietary patterns and potential impacts on JLI across cultures
2. Variations in stress levels and stress management practices worldwide
3. Global trends in physical activity and potential relations to JLI

12.12 Future Directions in Global JLI Management

Looking ahead to emerging trends and needs in worldwide JLI care.

12.12.1 Precision Medicine on a Global Scale

Tailoring treatments to diverse populations:

1. Challenges in developing personalized approaches for varied genetic backgrounds
2. Potential for global pharmacogenomic studies to inform treatment selections
3. Ethical considerations in implementing precision medicine across different healthcare systems

12.12.2 Artificial Intelligence and Global Diagnosis

Potential for AI to improve global JLI care:

1. Development of AI algorithms for JLI diagnosis trained on diverse global datasets
2. Use of AI to support clinical decision-making in resource-limited

settings

3. Ethical and practical challenges in implementing AI tools worldwide

12.12.3 Sustainable and Equitable Global Care Models

Striving for improved JLI management worldwide:

1. Developing sustainable models for providing specialized care in low-resource areas
2. Addressing global health disparities in JLI diagnosis and treatment
3. Balancing innovation with accessibility in future JLI management approaches

Conclusion

Jessner's Lymphocytic Infiltrate, while a relatively rare condition, presents a complex landscape of challenges and opportunities on a global scale. From variations in prevalence and presentation across different populations to disparities in healthcare access and resource availability, the global perspective on JLI is multifaceted and ever-evolving.

Key takeaways from this exploration of global perspectives and resources include:

1. The importance of understanding cultural, environmental, and healthcare system variations in approaching JLI management worldwide
2. The valuable role of international collaborations in advancing JLI research and care
3. The potential of telemedicine and digital health technologies to bridge gaps in global JLI care
4. The ongoing challenges in providing equitable, high-quality JLI man-

agement in resource-limited settings
5. The wealth of global resources available to support patients and healthcare providers in understanding and managing JLI

As we look to the future, the global management of Jessner's Lymphocytic Infiltrate will likely be shaped by advancements in precision medicine, artificial intelligence, and sustainable care models. However, the core principles of patient-centered care, evidence-based practice, and global health equity should remain at the forefront of these advancements.

By fostering international cooperation, leveraging technological innovations, and maintaining a commitment to equitable care, the global dermatology community can work towards improved outcomes for all individuals affected by JLI, regardless of their geographical location or socioeconomic circumstances. As our world becomes increasingly interconnected, so too must our approach to managing conditions like Jessner's Lymphocytic Infiltrate, ensuring that knowledge, resources, and high-quality care are accessible to all who need them.

CHAPTER 13

Research Frontiers and Future Directions

As our understanding of Jessner's Lymphocytic Infiltrate (JLI) continues to evolve, new avenues of research are constantly emerging. This chapter explores the cutting-edge research in JLI, ongoing clinical trials, and potential future directions that may revolutionize our approach to diagnosing, treating, and managing this condition.

13.1 Advances in Understanding JLI Pathogenesis

Recent years have seen significant progress in unraveling the underlying mechanisms of JLI.

13.1.1 Immunological Insights

Emerging research focuses on:
1. Characterization of T cell subsets involved in JLI lesions
   - Recent studies have identified specific T cell populations, including Th1 and Th17 cells, that may play crucial roles in JLI pathogenesis.
   - Investigation of regulatory T cell dysfunction as a potential contributing factor.

2. Role of innate immune responses
   - Exploration of the involvement of innate lymphoid cells (ILCs) in JLI.

- Studies on the contribution of neutrophils and mast cells to the inflammatory process.

3. Cytokine and chemokine profiles
- Identification of key inflammatory mediators, such as IFN-γ, TNF-α, and IL-17, in JLI lesions.
- Investigation of chemokine patterns that drive lymphocyte recruitment to the skin.

13.1.2 Genetic Studies

Ongoing genetic investigations include:
1. Genome-wide association studies (GWAS)
- Large-scale studies aiming to identify genetic loci associated with JLI susceptibility.
- Exploration of genetic variants that may influence disease severity or treatment response.

2. Epigenetic modifications
- Investigation of DNA methylation patterns and histone modifications in JLI lesions.
- Studies on the role of microRNAs in regulating gene expression in JLI.

3. Familial cases and hereditary components
- Detailed genetic analysis of familial JLI cases to identify potential heritable factors.
- Exploration of polygenic risk scores for predicting JLI susceptibility.

13.1.3 Environmental Triggers

Research into environmental factors involves:
1. UV radiation and JLI
- Molecular studies on UV-induced damage in JLI-prone skin.

- Investigation of photoprotective strategies specific to JLI patients.

2. Potential infectious triggers
   - Exploration of viral associations, including human herpesviruses and papillomaviruses.
   - Studies on the potential role of cutaneous microbiome dysbiosis in JLI pathogenesis.

3. Occupational and lifestyle factors
   - Investigation of occupational exposures that may increase JLI risk.
   - Studies on the impact of stress, diet, and other lifestyle factors on JLI development and progression.

13.2 Advances in Diagnostic Techniques

New diagnostic approaches are being developed to enhance accuracy and ease of JLI diagnosis.

13.2.1 Non-invasive Imaging Techniques

Promising technologies include:
   1. High-resolution optical coherence tomography (OCT)
   - Development of OCT protocols specific for JLI diagnosis and monitoring.
   - Studies comparing OCT findings with histopathological features of JLI.

2. Reflectance confocal microscopy (RCM)
   - Refinement of RCM criteria for differentiating JLI from other lymphocytic infiltrates.
   - Investigation of RCM as a tool for monitoring treatment response in JLI.

3. Multiphoton microscopy
   - Exploration of multiphoton imaging for assessing collagen and elastin changes in JLI lesions.

- Studies on the potential of multiphoton microscopy in differentiating JLI subtypes.

13.2.2 Biomarker Discovery

Ongoing research focuses on identifying:
1. Serum biomarkers
- Proteomic studies to identify circulating markers of JLI activity.
- Investigation of autoantibodies potentially associated with JLI.

2. Tissue biomarkers
- Immunohistochemical studies to identify specific markers of JLI in skin biopsies.
- Exploration of novel staining techniques to enhance diagnostic accuracy.

3. Genetic markers
- Development of genetic panels for assessing JLI risk or prognosis.
- Studies on pharmacogenomic markers to predict treatment response.

13.2.3 Artificial Intelligence in Diagnosis

Emerging applications of AI include:
1. Machine learning algorithms for clinical image analysis
- Development of AI models trained on large datasets of JLI clinical photographs.
- Studies on the accuracy of AI-assisted diagnosis compared to expert dermatologists.

2. AI-assisted histopathology
- Creation of deep learning models for analyzing JLI histopathological slides.
- Investigation of AI tools for quantifying inflammatory infiltrates in JLI biopsies.

3. Decision support tools
   - Development of AI-powered clinical decision support systems for JLI diagnosis and management.
   - Studies on the integration of AI tools into existing dermatology workflows.

13.3 Emerging Therapeutic Approaches

Novel treatment strategies are being explored to improve outcomes in JLI.

13.3.1 Targeted Immunotherapies

Promising areas of investigation include:
   1. JAK inhibitors
   - Clinical trials of topical and systemic JAK inhibitors in JLI.
   - Studies on the efficacy of selective JAK1 or JAK3 inhibitors in JLI management.

2. IL-23/IL-17 axis inhibitors
   - Investigation of IL-23 blockers (e.g., guselkumab, risankizumab) in JLI treatment.
   - Trials of IL-17 inhibitors (e.g., secukinumab, ixekizumab) for recalcitrant JLI.

3. Costimulation blockade agents
   - Exploration of abatacept and other T cell costimulation modulators in JLI.
   - Studies on the potential of targeting specific costimulatory pathways in JLI pathogenesis.

13.3.2 Biologics

Ongoing research on biologics focuses on:

1. Anti-TNF agents

- Long-term safety and efficacy studies of TNF inhibitors in JLI.

- Investigation of biosimilars as cost-effective alternatives for JLI treatment.

2. B cell-targeted therapies

- Exploration of rituximab and other B cell-depleting agents in refractory JLI.

- Studies on the role of B cells in JLI pathogenesis and as therapeutic targets.

3. Novel cytokine targets

- Investigation of agents targeting IL-1, IL-6, or other cytokines implicated in JLI.

- Exploration of bi-specific antibodies targeting multiple inflammatory pathways.

13.3.3 Small Molecule Inhibitors

Investigation of small molecule drugs includes:

1. Tyrosine kinase inhibitors

- Studies on the potential of BTK inhibitors in modulating B cell responses in JLI.

- Exploration of multi-kinase inhibitors for broad immunomodulation in JLI.

2. Phosphodiesterase inhibitors

- Clinical trials of topical and oral PDE4 inhibitors in JLI management.

- Investigation of novel PDE isoform-specific inhibitors for targeted therapy.

3. Proteasome inhibitors

- Exploration of bortezomib and next-generation proteasome inhibitors in severe JLI.

- Studies on the mechanisms of proteasome inhibition in modulating skin inflammation.

13.3.4 Cell-based Therapies

Emerging cellular approaches include:
1. Regulatory T cell (Treg) therapy
- Studies on ex vivo expansion and infusion of autologous Tregs in JLI.
- Investigation of methods to enhance Treg function in the skin.

2. Mesenchymal stem cell (MSC) therapy
- Exploration of MSC transplantation for immunomodulation in JLI.
- Studies on the paracrine effects of MSCs in skin inflammation.

3. Chimeric antigen receptor (CAR) T cell therapy
- Preliminary investigations into CAR-T cells targeting specific skin-homing T cell populations.
- Exploration of "off-the-shelf" CAR-T products for JLI treatment.

13.4 Advances in Drug Delivery and Formulation

Innovation in drug delivery systems aims to enhance treatment efficacy and patient compliance.

13.4.1 Nanotechnology-based Delivery

Emerging nanotechnology applications include:
1. Nanoparticle-based topical formulations
- Development of nanocarriers for enhanced skin penetration of JLI treatments.
- Studies on lipid nanoparticles for targeted delivery of immunomodulators.

2. Nanoengineered materials
   - Exploration of nanofiber scaffolds for controlled release of anti-inflammatory agents.
   - Investigation of "smart" nanoparticles responsive to skin inflammation.

3. Transdermal delivery systems
   - Development of microneedle patches for painless delivery of JLI medications.
   - Studies on iontophoresis and other physical methods to enhance drug penetration.

13.4.2 Novel Formulations

Research into improved drug formulations includes:
   1. Long-acting injectables
   - Development of depot formulations for sustained release of systemic JLI treatments.
   - Studies on the pharmacokinetics and efficacy of long-acting preparations.

2. Topical combination products
   - Investigation of fixed-dose combinations of corticosteroids and calcineurin inhibitors.
   - Exploration of novel vehicle technologies for improved skin penetration and tolerability.

3. Personalized formulations
   - Development of 3D-printed topical medications tailored to individual patient needs.
   - Studies on the use of artificial intelligence in optimizing formulation design.

13.5 Precision Medicine Approaches

The future of JLI management lies in personalized approaches tailored to individual patients.

13.5.1 Genetic Profiling

Advances in genetic analysis aim to:
   1. Identify genetic markers predictive of disease severity and progression
   - Large-scale genomic studies correlating genetic variants with JLI outcomes.
   - Development of polygenic risk scores for JLI prognosis.

2. Develop genetic tests to guide treatment selection
   - Pharmacogenomic studies to predict response to specific JLI therapies.
   - Investigation of rare genetic variants that may inform targeted treatment approaches.

3. Explore gene therapy approaches
   - Preliminary studies on gene editing techniques (e.g., CRISPR) in animal models of JLI.
   - Exploration of RNA interference therapies targeting key inflammatory mediators.

13.5.2 Immunophenotyping

Detailed immune profiling seeks to:
   1. Characterize individual patients' immune signatures
   - Single-cell RNA sequencing studies of JLI lesions to identify distinct cellular subpopulations.
   - Development of immune cell atlases specific to JLI.

2. Match specific immune profiles with optimal treatment strategies
   - Studies correlating immunophenotypes with response to different classes of therapy.

- Investigation of dynamic changes in immune profiles during JLI treatment.

3. Monitor immune responses to guide treatment adjustments
   - Development of minimally invasive methods for longitudinal immune monitoring.
   - Exploration of circulating immune cell populations as surrogate markers of skin inflammation.

13.5.3 Precision Medicine Algorithms

Development of decision support tools includes:
   1. Integration of clinical, genetic, and immunological data
   - Creation of comprehensive databases linking multi-omic data with clinical outcomes in JLI.
   - Development of AI-powered algorithms for treatment selection and prognosis prediction.

2. Machine learning models for predicting treatment outcomes
   - Large-scale studies applying machine learning to diverse datasets to improve predictive accuracy.
   - Investigation of deep learning approaches for analyzing complex patterns in JLI data.

3. Personalized risk stratification
   - Development of risk calculators incorporating multiple factors to guide JLI management.
   - Studies on the clinical implementation and validation of personalized risk tools.

13.6 Digital Health and Telemedicine Innovations

Emerging technologies are poised to transform JLI care in the digital age.

13.6.1 Smartphone-based Monitoring

Development of mobile health (mHealth) tools includes:

1. Apps for tracking JLI symptoms and treatment response
- Creation of validated digital instruments for patient-reported outcomes in JLI.
- Studies on the use of smartphone-based ecological momentary assessment in JLI research.

2. AI-powered skin imaging for home monitoring
- Development of smartphone apps using computer vision for assessing JLI lesions.
- Investigation of the accuracy and reliability of AI-assisted self-monitoring.

3. Integration with wearable devices
- Exploration of wearable sensors for continuous monitoring of skin parameters.
- Studies on the use of smartwatch data to predict JLI flares.

13.6.2 Telemedicine Platforms

Advancements in remote care delivery include:

1. High-resolution teledermatology systems
- Development of standardized imaging protocols for remote JLI assessment.
- Studies on the diagnostic accuracy of teledermatology compared to in-person evaluation.

2. Virtual reality (VR) applications
- Exploration of VR technologies for immersive patient education about JLI.
- Investigation of VR-assisted remote physical examinations.

3. Augmented reality (AR) in clinical practice
  - Development of AR tools to assist in precise topical treatment application.
  - Studies on AR-guided skin biopsy techniques for JLI diagnosis.

13.7 Psychodermatological Approaches

The integration of psychological and dermatological care continues to evolve.

13.7.1 Neuroimaging Studies

Investigations into the brain-skin connection include:
  1. Functional MRI studies of central nervous system responses in JLI
  - Exploration of neural correlates of itch and inflammation in JLI patients.
  - Studies on brain activation patterns in response to JLI treatments.

2. PET imaging of neuroinflammation
  - Investigation of neuroinflammatory processes potentially associated with JLI.
  - Exploration of the relationship between central and peripheral inflammation in JLI.

13.7.2 Psychoneuroimmunology

Research into mind-body interactions includes:
  1. Studies on stress-induced exacerbation of JLI
  - Investigation of neuroendocrine pathways linking stress to skin inflammation.
  - Exploration of the impact of psychological interventions on immune parameters in JLI.

2. Mindfulness-based interventions
  - Clinical trials of mindfulness meditation programs for JLI management.

- Studies on the neurobiological mechanisms underlying mindfulness effects in JLI.

13.7.3 Novel Psychological Therapies

Emerging approaches in psychodermatology include:
   1. Virtual reality therapy for body image concerns
   - Development of VR-based exposure therapy for JLI-related social anxiety.
   - Studies on the efficacy of VR interventions in improving quality of life in JLI patients.

2. Online cognitive-behavioral therapy (CBT) programs
   - Creation of JLI-specific digital CBT modules for scalable psychological support.
   - Investigation of the long-term outcomes of online CBT interventions in JLI management.

13.8 Translational Research Initiatives

Bridging the gap between basic science and clinical application is a key focus of current research.

13.8.1 Disease Modeling

Advanced approaches to studying JLI include:
   1. 3D skin organoids
   - Development of patient-derived skin organoids for personalized drug testing.
   - Studies using organoid models to investigate JLI pathogenesis and potential therapies.

2. Humanized mouse models
   - Creation of mouse models with human immune system components to

better mimic JLI.

- Exploration of xenograft models using patient-derived skin samples.

3. In silico modeling

- Development of computational models simulating JLI progression and treatment responses.

- Integration of multi-scale modeling approaches to understand complex JLI dynamics.

13.8.2 Bioengineering Approaches

Innovative research includes:

1. Skin-on-a-chip models

- Development of microfluidic devices mimicking skin structure and immune responses.

- Studies using skin-on-a-chip for high-throughput drug screening in JLI.

2. 3D bioprinting

- Exploration of 3D-printed skin equivalents for JLI research and drug testing.

- Investigation of bioprinted immune cell niches to study JLI pathogenesis.

Conclusion

The landscape of Jessner's Lymphocytic Infiltrate research is rapidly evolving, offering exciting prospects for improved understanding, diagnosis, and management of this challenging condition. From advances in basic science unraveling the pathogenesis of JLI to innovative clinical approaches and cutting-edge technologies, the future holds promise for significant improvements in patient care.

Key areas of future focus

CHAPTER 14

Ethical Considerations and Patient Advocacy in JLI Management

As our understanding and treatment of Jessner's Lymphocytic Infiltrate (JLI) continue to advance, it is crucial to consider the ethical implications of these developments and the role of patient advocacy in shaping the future of JLI care. This chapter explores the ethical challenges that arise in JLI research and management, as well as the growing importance of patient advocacy in driving progress and improving outcomes for those affected by this condition.

14.1 Ethical Considerations in JLI Research

The pursuit of scientific knowledge about JLI must be balanced with ethical considerations to protect patient rights and ensure responsible research practices.

14.1.1 Informed Consent in JLI Studies

Key ethical considerations include:
1. Ensuring comprehensive understanding
- Developing clear, accessible explanations of complex JLI research protocols
- Addressing language and cultural barriers in obtaining informed consent

2. Vulnerability and capacity
   - Protecting vulnerable populations in JLI research, including children and cognitively impaired individuals
   - Assessing capacity to consent in patients with severe or distressing JLI symptoms

3. Ongoing consent in longitudinal studies
   - Implementing processes for re-consenting participants in long-term JLI studies
   - Addressing changes in capacity over time, particularly in aging populations

14.1.2 Privacy and Confidentiality

Protecting patient information in the digital age:
   1. Data security in JLI registries and biobanks
   - Implementing robust encryption and access controls for sensitive patient data
   - Developing protocols for secure sharing of de-identified data in collaborative research

2. Genetic privacy concerns
   - Addressing the implications of genetic testing in JLI for patients and their families
   - Developing policies for handling incidental findings in genetic studies

3. Digital health and telemedicine considerations
   - Ensuring privacy in remote monitoring and teledermatology applications for JLI
   - Addressing cross-border data transfer issues in international JLI research

14.1.3 Ethical Use of Placebo Controls

Balancing scientific rigor with patient welfare:

1. Justification for placebo use in JLI trials
   - Evaluating the ethical acceptability of placebo controls in different JLI study designs
   - Considering alternative trial designs to minimize placebo use in vulnerable populations

2. Rescue treatments and early stopping rules
   - Implementing protocols for providing active treatment to placebo group participants if needed
   - Developing clear criteria for early termination of trials based on efficacy or safety concerns

3. Post-trial access to treatments
   - Ensuring continued access to effective treatments for study participants after trial completion
   - Addressing equity issues in providing post-trial care, particularly in resource-limited settings

14.2 Ethical Challenges in JLI Management

The clinical management of JLI presents its own set of ethical dilemmas that healthcare providers must navigate.

14.2.1 Off-label Use of Medications

Balancing innovation with patient safety:

1. Informed decision-making
   - Providing comprehensive information about potential risks and benefits of off-label treatments
   - Documenting discussions and obtaining explicit consent for off-label use in JLI

2. Evidence-based practice
- Developing guidelines for appropriate off-label prescribing in JLI management
- Encouraging systematic data collection and reporting of off-label treatment outcomes

3. Equity and access considerations
- Addressing disparities in access to off-label treatments due to cost or insurance coverage
- Balancing individual patient needs with resource allocation in healthcare systems

14.2.2 Personalized Medicine and Resource Allocation

Ethical implications of advanced diagnostic and treatment approaches:
1. Equitable access to precision medicine
- Addressing potential disparities in access to genetic testing and targeted therapies
- Developing policies for fair allocation of high-cost personalized treatments

2. Predictive testing and psychological impact
- Providing appropriate counseling and support for patients undergoing predictive genetic testing for JLI
- Addressing the ethical implications of identifying genetic risk in asymptomatic family members

3. Data ownership and commercialization
- Developing frameworks for responsible use of patient data in developing personalized therapies
- Addressing issues of benefit-sharing when patient data leads to commercial developments

14.2.3 End-of-Life Considerations in Severe JLI

Ethical challenges in managing refractory cases:
   1. Quality of life assessments
   - Developing tools to objectively assess quality of life in severe JLI cases
   - Integrating patient values and preferences into treatment decision-making

2. Palliative care approaches
   - Incorporating palliative care principles in managing distressing symptoms of advanced JLI
   - Addressing cultural and religious considerations in end-of-life care for JLI patients

3. Advance care planning
   - Encouraging early discussions about treatment preferences and goals of care
   - Developing JLI-specific advance directive tools to guide care in severe cases

14.3 Patient Advocacy in JLI

Patient advocacy plays a crucial role in driving progress in JLI research, treatment, and policy.

14.3.1 Role of Patient Advocacy Organizations

Key functions of JLI advocacy groups:
   1. Education and awareness
   - Developing and disseminating accurate, accessible information about JLI
   - Organizing awareness campaigns to increase public understanding of the condition

2. Research advocacy
   - Promoting patient-centered research priorities in JLI
   - Facilitating patient involvement in study design and implementation

3. Policy and legislation
   - Advocating for policies to improve access to JLI treatments and support services
   - Engaging with policymakers to address issues affecting the JLI community

14.3.2 Patient Engagement in Research

Enhancing the relevance and impact of JLI studies:
   1. Patient-reported outcomes
   - Developing and validating patient-reported outcome measures specific to JLI
   - Incorporating patient perspectives in defining meaningful endpoints for clinical trials

2. Patient and public involvement (PPI) in research design
   - Establishing frameworks for meaningful patient involvement throughout the research process
   - Training researchers in effective engagement with patient partners

3. Citizen science initiatives
   - Developing platforms for patient-led data collection and analysis in JLI research
   - Exploring the potential of crowdsourcing approaches to accelerate JLI discoveries

14.3.3 Empowering Patient Voices

Strategies for amplifying patient perspectives:

1. Patient advisory boards
- Establishing patient advisory boards within healthcare institutions and research organizations
- Ensuring diverse representation to capture the full spectrum of JLI experiences

2. Narrative medicine and patient stories
- Promoting the use of patient narratives in medical education and public awareness
- Developing platforms for patients to share their JLI journeys and insights

3. Social media and online communities
- Leveraging social media platforms to connect JLI patients and amplify their voices
- Addressing challenges of misinformation and maintaining privacy in online patient communities

14.4 Ethical Considerations in Global JLI Management

Addressing ethical challenges in managing JLI across diverse global contexts.

14.4.1 Cultural Competence and Respect

Ensuring culturally appropriate care:
1. Cultural sensitivity in diagnosis and treatment
- Developing culturally adapted assessment tools and treatment protocols for JLI
- Training healthcare providers in cultural competence specific to dermatological care

2. Respecting traditional healing practices
- Exploring ethical ways to integrate traditional medicines with evidence-based JLI treatments

- Addressing potential conflicts between cultural practices and medical recommendations

3. Language and communication
- Ensuring availability of qualified medical interpreters for JLI care in diverse populations
- Developing multilingual patient education materials and consent forms

14.4.2 Global Health Equity in JLI Care

Addressing disparities in JLI management worldwide:
1. Access to essential medications
- Advocating for inclusion of JLI treatments in national essential medicine lists
- Exploring innovative pricing models to improve access to high-cost therapies in low-resource settings

2. Capacity building in dermatology care
- Developing sustainable training programs to increase dermatology expertise in underserved regions
- Implementing teledermatology initiatives to extend specialist JLI care to remote areas

3. Research equity and benefit sharing
- Ensuring fair participation of low- and middle-income countries in JLI clinical trials
- Developing frameworks for equitable sharing of benefits from global JLI research

14.4.3 Ethical Challenges in International Collaborations

Navigating ethical issues in global JLI research:
1. Harmonizing ethical standards

- Developing consensus guidelines for ethical conduct of multinational JLI studies

- Addressing variations in regulatory requirements across different countries

2. Capacity building for ethical review
- Strengthening local ethics committee capabilities in reviewing JLI research protocols
- Promoting collaboration between ethics committees in high- and low-resource settings

3. Addressing power imbalances
- Ensuring equitable partnerships between researchers from different countries
- Developing mechanisms for fair authorship and recognition in international JLI publications

14.5 Ethical Implications of Emerging Technologies in JLI Care

Considering the ethical challenges posed by new technologies in JLI diagnosis and management.

14.5.1 Artificial Intelligence and Machine Learning

Ethical considerations in AI-assisted JLI care:
1. Algorithmic bias and fairness
- Addressing potential biases in AI algorithms trained on non-diverse JLI datasets
- Developing frameworks for fair and equitable implementation of AI in clinical decision-making

2. Transparency and explainability
- Ensuring interpretability of AI-based diagnostic and treatment recom-

mendations for JLI
- Developing guidelines for communicating AI-assisted decisions to patients

3. Accountability and liability
- Clarifying legal and ethical responsibilities in cases of AI-related errors in JLI management
- Developing protocols for ongoing monitoring and validation of AI systems in clinical use

14.5.2 Digital Health and Telemedicine

Ethical challenges in remote JLI care:
1. Digital divide and access disparities
- Addressing inequities in access to digital health technologies for JLI management
- Developing strategies to ensure quality care for patients without access to advanced technologies

2. Data privacy and security
- Implementing robust safeguards for patient data in telemedicine and remote monitoring applications
- Addressing cross-border data transfer issues in international telemedicine consultations

3. Quality of care and professional boundaries
- Developing standards for ensuring quality of care in telemedicine-based JLI management
- Addressing challenges in maintaining appropriate provider-patient relationships in virtual care settings

14.5.3 Gene Editing and Advanced Therapies

Ethical implications of cutting-edge JLI treatments:

1. Safety and long-term effects

- Developing robust long-term follow-up protocols for patients receiving gene therapies for JLI

- Addressing ethical challenges in first-in-human trials of advanced therapies

2. Germline modifications

- Exploring the ethical implications of potential germline interventions to prevent hereditary forms of JLI

- Developing international guidelines on the permissible uses of gene editing in JLI research and treatment

3. Enhancement and non-therapeutic uses

- Addressing ethical concerns about potential non-therapeutic applications of JLI-related genetic technologies

- Developing frameworks for distinguishing between treatment and enhancement in genetic interventions

14.6 The Future of Ethical JLI Management

Looking ahead to emerging ethical challenges and opportunities in JLI care.

14.6.1 Anticipatory Ethics

Proactively addressing future ethical issues:

1. Horizon scanning

- Establishing mechanisms to identify and address emerging ethical challenges in JLI research and care

- Engaging diverse stakeholders in anticipatory ethical deliberations

2. Ethical impact assessments

- Developing frameworks for assessing the ethical implications of new JLI

technologies and treatments
  - Integrating ethical considerations into the early stages of research and development processes

3. Adaptive governance
  - Creating flexible ethical guidelines that can evolve with advancing JLI knowledge and technologies
  - Implementing mechanisms for ongoing ethical oversight and policy adaptation

14.6.2 Empowering Ethical Decision-Making

Enhancing ethical competence in JLI management:
  1. Ethics education for healthcare providers
  - Integrating JLI-specific ethical training into dermatology and primary care curricula
  - Developing continuing education programs on emerging ethical issues in JLI care

2. Patient empowerment in ethical decisions
  - Developing decision aids to support patients in navigating complex ethical choices in JLI management
  - Promoting shared decision-making models that explicitly address ethical considerations

3. Ethical consultation services
  - Establishing specialized ethics consultation services for complex JLI cases
  - Developing networks for sharing ethical expertise across healthcare institutions

14.6.3 Global Ethical Framework for JLI

Towards a unified approach to ethical JLI management:

1. International consensus building

- Facilitating global dialogues to develop shared ethical principles for JLI research and care

- Addressing cultural and contextual variations in ethical norms while striving for core universal standards

2. Integrating ethics into global health initiatives

- Incorporating ethical considerations into international JLI research collaborations and capacity-building efforts

- Developing ethical guidelines for global health interventions targeting JLI and related skin conditions

3. Ethical innovation in resource-limited settings

- Exploring innovative, ethically sound approaches to improving JLI care in low-resource environments

- Promoting ethical research and development of affordable, accessible JLI treatments for global use

Conclusion

The ethical landscape of Jessner's Lymphocytic Infiltrate management is complex and evolving, reflecting the broader challenges in dermatology and healthcare at large. As we advance in our understanding and treatment of JLI, it is crucial to maintain a strong ethical foundation that respects patient autonomy, ensures equitable access to care, and promotes responsible research practices.

The role of patient advocacy in shaping the future of JLI care cannot be overstated. By amplifying patient voices, promoting patient-centered research, and advocating for policies that improve the lives of those affected by JLI, advocacy efforts play a vital role in driving progress and ensuring that advancements in JLI management truly meet the needs of patients.

As we look to the future, the integration of ethical considerations into all aspects of JLI research, care, and policy development will be essential. By fostering a culture of ethical reflection and dialogue, we can navigate the challenges ahead and work towards a future where JLI management is not only scientifically advanced but also ethically sound and truly patient-centered.

CONCLUSION

The Future of Jessner's Lymphocytic Infiltrate Management

As we conclude this comprehensive exploration of Jessner's Lymphocytic Infiltrate (JLI), it is clear that we stand at a pivotal moment in our understanding and management of this complex dermatological condition. Throughout this book, we have traversed the landscape of JLI from its historical foundations to the cutting-edge research shaping its future. Now, we will synthesize these insights and look ahead to the challenges and opportunities that lie before us in the field of JLI care.

Reflecting on Our Journey

Our exploration began with the historical context and basic science underpinning JLI. We delved into the intricate immunological mechanisms at play, unraveling the complex interplay between T cells, cytokines, and other immune mediators that contribute to the characteristic lymphocytic infiltrate. This foundational knowledge has proven crucial in understanding the pathogenesis of JLI and in developing targeted therapeutic approaches.

We then navigated the clinical landscape of JLI, examining its varied presentations, diagnostic challenges, and management strategies. The importance of accurate diagnosis, often requiring careful clinicopathological correlation, was emphasized. We explored the range of treatment modalities available, from topical therapies to systemic medications and phototherapy, highlighting the need for individualized treatment plans tailored to each patient's unique presentation and circumstances.

Our journey took us through the lived experiences of individuals with JLI, shedding light on the profound impact this condition can have on quality of life, psychological well-being, and social interactions. These patient perspectives serve as a powerful reminder of the human element at the heart of our scientific and clinical endeavors.

We examined JLI through various lenses – considering its presentation in special populations, exploring global perspectives, and delving into the ethical considerations that arise in research and clinical practice. The complexity of managing JLI across diverse cultural, geographical, and healthcare contexts became evident, underscoring the need for flexible, culturally sensitive approaches to care.

Finally, we ventured into the frontiers of JLI research, exploring emerging technologies, novel therapeutic approaches, and the promise of precision medicine. The rapid pace of scientific advancement in fields such as immunology, genetics, and artificial intelligence holds tremendous potential for revolutionizing JLI management in the coming years.

Current State of JLI Management

As it stands today, the management of JLI remains challenging, often requiring a combination of therapeutic approaches and long-term follow-up. While we have made significant strides in understanding the immunological basis of JLI and in developing more targeted treatments, many patients still struggle with recalcitrant disease or cycles of remission and relapse.

The current treatment landscape offers a range of options, from topical corticosteroids and calcineurin inhibitors to systemic medications like antimalarials and immunosuppressants. Phototherapy continues to play a significant role, with modalities like narrowband UVB showing efficacy in many cases. However, the variability in treatment response and the potential for side effects with long-term use of some therapies remain ongoing challenges.

Diagnostic accuracy has improved with advances in immunohistochemistry and the growing recognition of JLI's distinctive features. However, the overlap with other lymphocytic skin disorders still presents diagnostic dilemmas in some cases, highlighting the need for continued refinement of our diagnostic criteria and tools.

The importance of a holistic approach to JLI management has become increasingly recognized. This encompasses not only medical treatments but also psychological support, lifestyle modifications, and patient education. The growing emphasis on patient-reported outcomes and quality of life measures reflects a more patient-centered approach to care.

Emerging Trends and Future Directions

As we look to the future, several key trends and directions are likely to shape the landscape of JLI management:

1. Precision Medicine: The advent of sophisticated genetic and immunological profiling techniques promises to usher in an era of more personalized treatment for JLI. By identifying specific genetic markers or immune signatures associated with different disease subtypes or treatment responses, we may be able to tailor therapies more precisely to individual patients.

2. Targeted Biologics: The success of biologic therapies in other dermatological conditions has spurred interest in their potential for JLI. As our understanding of the specific cytokine pathways involved in JLI pathogenesis deepens, we can anticipate the development of more targeted biologic therapies that may offer improved efficacy with fewer side effects.

3. Artificial Intelligence and Digital Health: The integration of AI into dermatological practice is likely to transform JLI diagnosis and management. From AI-assisted image analysis for more accurate diagnosis to machine learning algorithms predicting treatment outcomes, these technologies hold the potential to enhance clinical decision-making and patient care.

4. Telemedicine and Remote Monitoring: The rapid adoption of telemedicine, accelerated by recent global events, is likely to have lasting impacts on JLI care. Remote consultations, teledermatology platforms, and digital tools for patient monitoring may improve access to specialist care and enable more continuous disease management.

5. Microbiome Research: Growing interest in the role of the skin microbiome in dermatological conditions may open new avenues for JLI management. Understanding how the microbiome interacts with the immune system in JLI could lead to novel therapeutic approaches, potentially including probiotic or prebiotic interventions.

6. Advanced Drug Delivery Systems: Innovations in drug delivery, such as nanoparticle-based formulations or 3D-printed medications, may enhance the efficacy of existing treatments and enable the development of new therapeutic strategies for JLI.

7. Psychodermatological Approaches: The increasing recognition of the bidirectional relationship between skin and mind is likely to lead to more integrated approaches combining dermatological and psychological interventions for comprehensive JLI management.

Challenges Ahead

Despite these promising directions, several challenges lie ahead in advancing JLI care:

1. Heterogeneity of Disease: The variability in JLI presentation and treatment response continues to pose challenges for developing standardized management protocols. Further research is needed to understand the factors underlying this heterogeneity and to develop more nuanced classification systems.

2. Long-term Safety of Treatments: As patients with JLI often require long-term management, ensuring the safety of prolonged treatment regimens remains a critical concern. Continued vigilance and long-term follow-up studies will be essential.

3. Access and Equity: Ensuring equitable access to advanced diagnostic tools and novel therapies for JLI patients worldwide presents significant challenges. Addressing disparities in care across different healthcare systems and socioeconomic contexts will be crucial.

4. Research Funding: As a relatively rare condition, securing adequate funding for JLI research can be challenging. Advocacy efforts and collaborations will be important in ensuring continued investment in JLI studies.

5. Ethical Considerations: The advent of genetic technologies and AI in healthcare brings with it a host of ethical considerations that will need to be carefully navigated in JLI management.

The Path Forward

To address these challenges and capitalize on emerging opportunities, several key strategies will be important:

1. Collaborative Research Networks: Fostering international collaborations and establishing robust research networks will be crucial for advancing our understanding of JLI. Multicenter studies and data sharing initiatives can help overcome the limitations posed by the rarity of the condition.

2. Patient-Centered Approach: Continuing to prioritize patient perspectives and experiences in research and clinical practice will be essential. This includes further development of patient-reported outcome measures and increased involvement of patient advocates in setting research priorities.

3. Interdisciplinary Collaboration: Given the complex nature of JLI, fostering collaboration between dermatologists, immunologists, geneticists, psychologists, and other specialists will be key to developing comprehensive management strategies.

4. Translational Research: Strengthening the pipeline from basic science discoveries to clinical applications will be crucial for developing new therapies. This includes investment in translational research infrastructure and support for early-phase clinical trials.

5. Education and Training: Ensuring that healthcare providers are well-equipped to diagnose and manage JLI will require ongoing education efforts. This includes updating medical curricula and providing continuing education opportunities to keep pace with rapidly advancing knowledge.

6. Global Health Perspective: Addressing JLI from a global health perspective, considering diverse healthcare contexts and cultural factors, will be important for developing universally applicable management strategies.

A Call to Action

As we conclude this comprehensive exploration of Jessner's Lymphocytic Infiltrate, it is clear that while significant progress has been made, much work remains to be done. To the researchers, clinicians, patients, and advocates engaged in the field of JLI, this book serves not only as a resource but also as a call to action.

For researchers, the challenge is to push the boundaries of our understanding, leveraging new technologies and interdisciplinary approaches to unravel the complexities of JLI pathogenesis and to develop innovative therapeutic strategies.

For clinicians, the task is to stay abreast of rapidly evolving knowledge, to approach each patient with a personalized and holistic perspective, and to contribute to the collective understanding through careful observation and documentation of clinical experiences.

For patients and advocates, your voices and experiences are invaluable in shaping the future of JLI research and care. Continued engagement, from participating in clinical trials to advocating for research funding and policy changes, is crucial in driving progress.

Looking Ahead with Hope

As we stand at this juncture in the history of JLI management, there is much cause for optimism. The rapid pace of scientific advancement, the growing emphasis on patient-centered care, and the increasing global collaboration in dermatological research all point towards a future where JLI can be more effectively managed, and perhaps one day, prevented or cured.

The journey of understanding and managing Jessner's Lymphocytic Infiltrate is far from over. It is a journey that will require continued dedication, innovation, and collaboration from all stakeholders in the dermatology community and beyond. As we move forward, let us carry with us the insights gained from the past, the knowledge of the present, and a vision for a future where JLI no longer poses a significant burden to those affected by it.

In closing, it is our hope that this book has not only provided a comprehensive overview of the current state of JLI knowledge but also inspired new questions, sparked innovative ideas, and reinforced the commitment to improving the lives of individuals affected by this challenging condition. The future of JLI management is in our hands, and together, we can work towards a world where Jessner's Lymphocytic Infiltrate is no longer a mystery, but a manageable and perhaps even preventable condition.

www.ingramcontent.com/pod-product-compliance
Lightning Source LLC
Chambersburg PA
CBHW070825250726
48662CB00003B/1093